T0270523

# Raising
# Healthy
# Kids

# Raising Healthy Kids

## Protecting Your Children from Hidden Chemical Toxins

David Steinman

author of the bestselling *Diet for a Poisoned Planet*
founder of the Healthy Living Foundation

Foreword by Sharon C. Lavigne
Winner of the 2021 Goldman Environmental Prize

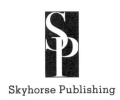

Skyhorse Publishing

The information provided in this book is designed to provide accurate and authoritative information with respect to the subject matter covered. This book is not meant to be used, nor should it be used, to diagnose or treat any medical condition. For diagnosis or treatment of any medical problem, consult your own physician. While every attempt is made to provide accurate information, the authors or publisher cannot be held accountable for any errors, omissions, or material which is no longer up to date.

Copyright © 2024 by David Steinman
Foreword copyright © 2024 by Sharon C. Lavigne

All rights reserved. No part of this book may be reproduced in any manner without the express written consent of the publisher, except in the case of brief excerpts in critical reviews or articles. All inquiries should be addressed to Skyhorse Publishing, 307 West 36th Street, 11th Floor, New York, NY 10018.

Skyhorse Publishing books may be purchased in bulk at special discounts for sales promotion, corporate gifts, fund-raising, or educational purposes. Special editions can also be created to specifications. For details, contact the Special Sales Department, Skyhorse Publishing, 307 West 36th Street, 11th Floor, New York, NY 10018 or info@skyhorsepublishing.com.

Skyhorse® and Skyhorse Publishing® are registered trademarks of Skyhorse Publishing, Inc.®, a Delaware corporation.

Visit our website at www.skyhorsepublishing.com.

10 9 8 7 6 5 4 3 2 1

Library of Congress Cataloging-in-Publication Data is available on file.

Cover design by David Ter-Avanesyan
Jacket photographs by iStock; apple by Getty Images
Interior illustrations by Getty Images

Print ISBN: 978-1-5107-7439-1
Ebook ISBN: 978-1-5107-7440-7

Printed in the United States of America

*To my children,*
*Spenser Blake, Hunter Hawkins, Sharla Rose,*
*and all children.*
*And to all the parents doing their best*
*to raise healthy kids.*

# Table of Contents

# Foreword

by Sharon C. Lavigne

2021 Goldman Environmental Prize Winner

I live where chemical and industrial plants crowd eighty-five miles of riverbanks along the Mississippi between Baton Rouge and New Orleans in a region of Louisiana known as Cancer Alley. Not surprisingly, we suffer the highest incidence of cancer here in the nation, according to the Environmental Protection Agency.

My family roots here go back two hundred years. Some of my ancestors were enslaved here. Others, like my mother and father, grew up here as free women and men who wanted nothing more than to raise healthy children. We grew vegetables in our garden, raised cattle, pigs, and hens, and baked pecan pie from the nuts of our own trees. My grandpa netted fish and shrimp from the river. I raised six children here. They blessed me by twelve.

I started teaching special education for the local school district in 1982. Things had already begun to change in the 1960s, however, when the chemical plants came. By the time I was teaching in the 1980s, the number of special-education students in my classroom had begun to grow at a much faster rate. Now I understand why. All around us, day and night, plants emit chemical toxins that pollute our air, water, food, and even our children. Nighttime chemical releases causing toxic "yellow rain" and burning orange flares of poisonous fumes are common. Our drinking water is contaminated with chemicals that cause cancer and reproductive harm.

In April 2018, Formosa, a multinational plastic group based in Taiwan, proposed construction of a new nine-billion-dollar chemical plant in St. James Parish, where I live, that would release hundreds of tons of chemical toxins into our community, not to mention exacerbate global climate change.

Our local parish council thought, since we are a predominantly Black community, we wouldn't rise in opposition when they gave approval.

They didn't know us—or our resolve.

I wasn't always an activist. However, I drew on the memories and stories of my mother and father's own civil rights activism and began organizing just like they would have done and urged me to do.

I held meetings at my home until we needed more space and moved to larger and larger places. I shared facts about the environment and cancer. Local folks shared stories about their family health issues. We invited experts to speak to us about the toxic effects of the chemicals to which we are being exposed.

EarthJustice, the nonprofit legal group, represented our community in federal court and, in a landmark case, Judge Trudy White revoked the company's permits on environmental justice grounds.

It was a powerful victory for the people—so far. The state of Louisiana plans to build or expand more than another one hundred petrochemical facilities in and around Cancer Alley. We are literally in a life and death battle here.

Needless to say, it's dangerous for a child growing up here. And it's even more difficult and heartbreaking for parents who desperately want to raise healthy kids. It's like an entire area of children's health is being ignored not only here in this region but across our nation. It's not taught in the schools. Doctors don't tell us about it. But protecting our kids from hidden chemical toxins is as important as knowing about nutrition or dental hygiene. Maybe even more important!

Most people, whether from the government or media, when they come to visit, stay a few hours, take a quick tour, and return to dine and lodge in New Orleans.

The author of this book, David Steinman, came to our community many times. He stayed at the local motels where all you see are pickup trucks with license plates of workers who come here from Texas, Arkansas, Mississippi, and other southern states to work in the chemical plants. They live for the week at the motels, doing their assigned shifts, getting exposed to chemical toxins, then return home. David woke up in the morning and smelled the fumes, saw the plumes of carcinogens puff like poisoned cotton balls into the air, and tasted, along with my family, the often unfit-to-drink water we have to imbibe daily. It was his mission, he said, to make sure what he wrote in *Raising Healthy Kids* could be used by everyone—no matter where they lived or what their budget.

I mentioned how some folks in Cancer Alley may make seventeen thousand dollars—in a good year. He shipped us water pitcher filters when he learned that what pours from our taps contains cancerous chemicals like atrazine and another one known as HEX that causes kidney and liver damage. He said that doing simple things like filtering our water costs less than thirty dollars and could be more important to family health than the best medical insurance policy around.

Then he went with me, up and down the river, where I showed him all of the nearby homes where there's cancer in the families.

We went to visit the ancient gravesite of the enslaved on the old Buena Vista Plantation where Formosa wants to build its plastics plant and even drew the ire of a local private security guard who didn't want us to pay our respects.

Another time, he wanted to meet the children of the Fifth Ward Elementary School in nearby Reserve, Louisiana, and arranged for a meeting with Principal Rajean Butler along with Robert Taylor, founder of Concerned Citizens of St. John the Baptist, myself, and others. The kids there are being exposed to the carcinogen chloroprene, used to make Neoprene. The Federal Department of Justice (DOJ) has filed litigation against the nearby polluting plant in order to curb their wanton contamination. But that won't help the kids who are at the Fifth Ward school now. After meeting with the principal, we all worked together to fund high-efficiency particle air filters for the school to be placed in every classroom and teachers' meeting spaces. This would measurably reduce the kids' exposures to dangerous pollutants that can impact their health while activists, along with the DOJ, fight in court to curb this plant's emissions. This is the cleanest air the kids will breathe all day. I think it will make a big difference in their health and academic performance.

*Raising Healthy Kids* is like getting helpful advice from that loving older brother or your most trusted best friend who cares enough about you to share everything you need to know but won't get anywhere else.

In this illuminating book is powerful inspiration, information, and imagination. David makes everything clear and manageable—his writing empowers.

You can raise healthy kids, knowing that when you take care of your own family you are making communities safer across America, too.

I truly urge you to enjoy this story that will change your and your kids' lives forever and for the better.

# Introduction

# My Promise

I have three kids, two dogs, and one leopard gecko. I call them the hearts that beat outside my body. If you're reading this book, it's likely you have a heart or hearts beating outside your body too and, like me, go to bed every night with gratitude your kids are all right. I certainly do. I pray a lot they are okay. Not a moment passes when they aren't being held close in my thoughts if not my arms.

Kids face so many pressures today that never even existed when we were their age. Social media constantly amplifies the messages children receive. Puberty brings on hormonal surges, different feelings, and a new world of learning about gender identity, sexual attraction, and even greater peer pressure.[1]

To deal with these issues, kids are counseled by parents, teachers, and other professionals. We have free school lunches and the federal Supplemental Nutrition Assistance Program, also known as SNAP, to aid families and children.

All of these are meant to help and support our children. But there's another ever-present danger that impacts their health and parents know next to nothing about when it comes to protecting them: their increasing exposures to the everyday toxic, hidden chemicals in our lives. Everyone knows they harm kids. And companies frequently know about the harmful chemicals their products contain but won't share this information, instead covering up what you need to know.

I wrote *Raising Healthy Kids* for parents and anybody else who desires to become better informed about how to protect their children from the hidden chemical toxins in their everyday lives.

I know the importance of alerting the public to toxic dangers.

In 2012, I founded the nonprofit legal advocacy group Healthy Living Foundation (HLF), one of the primary enforcers of the California Safe Drinking Water and Toxic Enforcement Act (often called Prop. 65) the voters of the state passed in 1986 with a nearly two-thirds majority. The law requires disclosure of harmful chemicals in foods, water, air, and consumer products found at amounts that cause cancer or reproductive toxicity. It's the most citizen-empowering, effective consumer law in the nation, perhaps in the civilized world.

It's good for democracy and the power of the people. For once, it gives the people some power over corporations. The law applies only to products sold in California. But many companies offer the same products throughout the nation.

The HLF has won court-approved, legally binding consent judgments and publicly disclosed settlement agreements that have made companies like Bumble Bee, Chicken of the Sea, Procter & Gamble, Kroger, Walmart, and Patagonia label their products for industrial chemicals and heavy metals that cause cancer and reproductive harm with prominent warnings that are easy to read and comprehend.[2, 3, 4, 5, 6] These warnings must appear on the product and website (if sold online) in a conspicuous manner (sometimes in multiple languages) before shoppers purchase them.

From Scotchgard to Gore-Tex, from Tide to Mr. Clean, from Simple Green to Ralph Lauren, and even Johnson & Johnson's, the question of how the chemicals in these products affect your children's health has never been more important.

The good news is we can do something about this problem, protect our families, and create better laws, all in the course of becoming smarter shoppers and parents.

But you're not getting this information. Not at all. Leading up to and during pregnancy, expectant parents are told to avoid alcohol and cigarettes, to make sure they get enough folic acid and omega-3 fatty acids, adequate sleep, and exercise. Yet, they're never told anything about how to reduce their exposure to chemical toxins. These could have an even greater impact on their baby's health!

Doctors and health-care providers are often poorly educated when it comes to chemical toxins, not well-versed in environmental exposures, and unable to effectively help their patients.[7]

Yet, knowledge is power. Studies confirm the more we know about the hidden chemical toxins in everyday living, the more often we will be able to keep them out of our children's lives.[8]

*Raising Healthy Kids* will take you on a deep dive into multitudes of everyday items found where you live and your children go to school in order to guide you and your family safely through this world where toxic chemicals have more rights than our children.

I'm going to make things simple and direct. This powerful, results-oriented prescription, with its plentiful safe-shopping charts, will empower you to keep your family healthy; it will also show you the most important action steps to take, including how to do the following, to become your family's protective shield:

- **Reduce your children's toxic burden.** I'll share test results from HLF and other reliable sources (using independent, third-party-certified laboratories) to show you the safe brands for your kids and unsafe ones to avoid.
- **Afford organic foods.** People often tell me organic food is out of reach for their budget; this a myth. My cost-saving suggestions will make organic affordable on any budget.
- **Kick the worst snack brands to the curb.** You'll find all the dirt about Justin's, Chex, Earth's Best, Trader Joe's, and other major brands that put kids' health at risk.
- **Choose safe personal care and beauty products.** Parents and teens alike need to be educated about the fake estrogens and testosterone blockers circulating in beauty products and how to find safe alternatives. The HLF has performed numerous tests to reveal the most toxic brands to avoid and those that are safe.
- **Select least-toxic ethnic hair products.** Persons with kinky, wavy, frizzy, or curly hair need not despair. There's a whole new world of safe and effective hairstyling products just for us.
- **Protect kids from outdoor pollutants.** An industrial plant near your home could be emitting silent toxins that threaten your pregnancy or children. I'll show you a proven protection plan.
- **Buy safe cleaning products.** It's really as simple as reaching to your left instead of right when picking out a product from store shelves. I'll let you know which brands can be trusted.
- **Filter your tap and bathing water.** No hype here. I went to the actual peer-reviewed, published studies to discover the most effective filtration systems.
- **Follow the new school rules.** I'll reveal how to keep your kids safe from asbestos, pesticides, and other harmful chemicals when at school.
- **Prevent tracking pollution into your home with an inexpensive tip that costs nothing and will save cleaning time.** The weird thing is fewer than a third of Americans actually do this on a consistent basis.

- **Curb 5G pocket sperm killers.** I'll share indispensable tips parents need to know about how to keep kids from using their smartphones to do dumb things to themselves like harming their attention span or brain cells.
- **Make sense of the new normal.** Chemical toxins and fake estrogens are impacting all of our families. We need to know the facts and most advanced scientific findings about the biology of gender identity in order to raise healthy children.
- **End toxic insanity.** Instead of playing the endless game of chemical Whac-A-Mole where one bad compound gets replaced by another even less well-studied substance, we need a policy of zero tolerance and generation of powerful young activists. *Raising Healthy Kids* will show you how to help your children become environmentally aware, antitoxic activists and defenders of our planet.

The motto of the HLF is chemical toxins that cause cancer or reproductive harm must be completely removed from the marketplace. Industry-funded lawmakers and scientists say a little bit of this or that poison is okay. But they are gaslighting you. Carcinogens and reproductive toxins have no safe threshold. The only sound public health policy is their complete elimination. Anything short of zero tolerance will only keep this toxic trainload barreling down the tracks.

I have had the opportunity to work with activists, scientists, and legal experts using the law to prevent sickness before it happens by demanding companies either remove or disclose hidden harmful chemicals in their foods and consumer products. Children are most healthy when least exposed to harmful chemicals. But the information we have a right to know about is being kept from us.

Too many corporations feel it's a virtue to keep you in the dark. To me, it's a sin and why I've taken legal actions in court to force them with the law to reveal to you what they're trying to hide. That's why I'm writing this story.

I promise to shed light.

# Time to Eat!

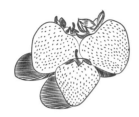
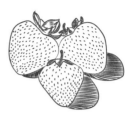

Chapter 1

# Organic Strawberry Fields Forever

"I grew up in a labor camp, and crop dusters used to be my morning alarm," Oscar Ramos, a second-grade teacher at the Sherwood Elementary School in the small agricultural town of Salinas, California, told me. "I used to go outside to see the planes and helicopters spray the fields across from where we lived. I thought it was 'cool,' but that's only because at such an early age I didn't know the dangers."

Most likely, when you sit down to dinner tonight, the moist and tender broccoli, cauliflower, Brussels sprouts, lettuce, and strawberries that nurture your body were planted and harvested by the parents of one of Oscar's students. The fields around this small town, situated at the northern end of the Salinas Valley, have long been known as the nation's salad bowl. The town is literally carved from the fields.

Today, raising his own adopted son, Manuel, with his wife, Kathleen, Oscar has taken the time to educate them about the harm pesticides can cause to their health. Records show each year before the pandemic more than five hundred thousand pounds of organophosphate (OP) pesticides alone, all powerful reproductive and nerve toxins, were applied to the crops in just this small region of the valley.[1]

Inspired by the late equal rights activist and labor leader Cesar Chavez, who visited Salinas and organized the local farm workers there into a viable union when he was a child, Oscar has learned a lot about living a healthy life and how to protect himself from the toxic effects pesticides seem to be having on his community. He holds educational workshops to share these lessons among his students and farmworker parents.

"I've been teaching in Salinas at the same school for twenty-five years," Oscar said. "I've seen the effects of pesticides used in our area and how they're taking a toll. Increasingly, especially in the last decade, we've been seeing more and more kids struggling in the classroom. Attention-deficit disorders are on the rise;

behavioral issues are getting worse. The inability and struggle of some students to make simple language, mathematical, and life connections in the classroom is increasingly visible. It's difficult and frustrating for teachers to see this and know it's largely irreversible, but I can only imagine how difficult and frustrating it is for my students themselves. I can see the tears in their faces when they look at me as if they're saying, 'I'm really trying, teacher, but I just don't understand.' It's heartbreaking to see them want to learn but be unable to comprehend or retain the lessons we are presenting. As teachers, we have to find multiple ways to reach these students, but it's taking an enormous toll on all of us."

The reason I have visited Salinas to start this story is the children here have become one of the most intensively studied populations in the world when it comes to understanding (and reducing) the toxic effects on our health from the chemicals in our diet, beauty products, and household cleaners. This is thanks to the work of Dr. Brenda Eskenazi, University of California (UC) Berkeley professor emeritus, and her colleagues, whose commitment to the health of the community began in the late 1990s with the Center for the Health Assessment of Mothers and Children of Salinas or CHAMACOS (Mexican slang for "children") study.

Pregnant women were recruited to participate from six community clinics between October 1999 and 2000. The researchers measured the amount of dialkyl phosphate (DAP)—a marker chemical that indicates exposure to OP pesticides—collected from the urine of expectant mothers during pregnancy and in their children at six months through age five. Their kids have been studied ever since so that we can know everything possible about how the OP pesticides have impacted their lives.

The work of Dr. Eskenazi, her team, and the selfless contributions of these six hundred moms and the CHAMACOS kids themselves is so important, far-ranging, and deserving of national attention that I will revisit their community throughout this book.

Daisy Gallardo, now twenty-two and a graduate of UC Berkeley, is one of the CHAMACOS children. When Daisy was five, she and the other study kids were administered the Wechsler Intelligence Scale for Children, the gold standard for measuring cognitive ability including verbal comprehension, visual spatial abilities, fluid reasoning, working memory, and processing speed. Her first memories of her involvement in the study involved "going to a fancy doctor's office for an appointment, playing computer games, and getting prizes. I didn't know what it was all about then, of course. But now I know these were tests being administered to measure various markers of our cognitive development."

Later, as a teen, Daisy recalls visiting medical offices again and having a "cap" placed over her skull for the specialist to perform neuroimaging to see how much of her cortical brain tissue was fully or only partially developed.

The results were startling and sobering. The CHAMACOS kids with the highest OP pesticide exposures had an average deficit of seven IQ points compared to the least exposed.[2] Those children also experienced increased incidence of attention deficit/hyperactivity disorder (ADHD).[3] The toxic effects "were stronger in boys," according to the study. As for those strange skullcaps the kids wore for follow-up neuroimaging, the most pesticide-exposed children had less brain capacity and working cortical tissue; the damage appeared permanent.[4]

In a simple twist of fate, however, Daisy might have been spared some of the worst exposures during her mother's pregnancy. Daisy's mom, Virginia, and dad, Onesimo, are farmworkers in the lettuce fields of Salinas. Their hand-weeding jobs, currently being replaced by the use of auto thinners that spray chemical herbicides, spared them some of the worst toxic exposures. If they'd been working in the fields with auto thinners, her mom's exposure to pesticides during pregnancy would, no doubt, have been higher.

Daisy recalls friends, some in the study, who weren't as fortunate. "They seemed really smart but leveled off with grade school," she said. "Like they couldn't go any farther. There were a lot more gangs and shootings when the pesticide use was at its worst. Maybe it's just a correlation, but I think if we had less spraying, many of the kids I grew up with could have accomplished more. But, I've learned from the study to be careful about the foods I buy, especially because I want to take better care of my parents as they get older and make sure my family stays healthy. I'm looking for a lot more organic foods."

Oh, you say you don't live in Salinas? So, what could these rural kids' health issues have to do with your children? Three thousand miles away, researchers at the Columbia Center for Children's Environmental Health in New York City have found urban kids from Harlem and the South Bronx suffer the same OP pesticide-related brain damage, including loss of cortical mass, IQ, and working memory as the most highly exposed CHAMACOS youth.[5, 6]

How is it these city kids are as bad off? The answer can be found strolling down the produce aisles of your local supermarket. All those inviting and blemish-free Brussels sprouts, broccoli, and heads of lettuce are more awash than ever with pesticide residues.[7] The US Food and Drug Administration (FDA) says more than 60 percent of our domestic produce has one or more pesticide residues. Tests of imported food items found more than half contained one or more pesticides. More than 3 percent of domestic food samples and almost 12 percent of imports have pesticide residues above our already ineffectual legal limits.

But it's actually far worse than this. Together, the FDA and California pesticide-monitoring reports—supplemented with published, peer-reviewed studies, and independent testing by the Healthy Living Foundation (HLF), the group for which I am chief officer—provide unsettling evidence of a toxic dietary mess.[8] But you don't have to be part of this insanity. You can become part of the solution and make sure your kids stay healthy.

## Organic Strawberry Fields Forever— A Family Protection Plan

The low-toxin diet and lifestyle I'll detail throughout *Raising Healthy Kids* helps flush out past toxic exposures, allowing the body to begin its own healing process.

The results we see with the switch to an organic diet are spectacular. Levels of pesticides measured in your blood, fatty tissues, and urine will be reduced, which will lead to strong improvements in your health—and your children's—with less risk for cancer, diabetes, obesity, miscarriages, brain fog, and pregnancy complications.[9, 10, 11, 12]

In the low-toxin diet, two-thirds of all servings of your foods, especially fruits and vegetables, should be organic, which means they were grown without the use of harmful synthetic pesticides or fertilizers. Organic farmers rely instead on least-toxic methods such as beneficial insects including lacewings and nematodes, hand-weeding, and biodegradable fatty-acid soaps. In contrast, conventional produce is grown with phosphate- and nitrate-rich fertilizers, which pollute our rivers and estuaries, and sprayed with pesticides that cause cancer and are toxic to the fetus.

It's critical to make as much of your produce as organic as possible. That is because veggies, fruits, seeds, nuts, and grains form the foundation of a healthy diet but are most likely to contain fresh residues of the OP pesticides that are so toxic to growing children. On the other hand, every California monitoring report and other studies I've reviewed, including the most recent from Europe, show organics to be largely free from them.[13] Be sure to look for the United States Department of Agriculture  certified seal when you do shop organics.

## *Organics on a Budget*

Don't fret. You don't need to be perfect either. Just two-thirds of your food choices should be organic to lower your toxin levels and improve your child's health, according to the studies.

I've done extensive online and in-store comparative price shopping to put together a comprehensive guide to show you safe and unsafe choices and how to make organics affordable.

Being a journalist and activist, I also know what it's like to raise one's family on a budget and shop for bargains at the dollar stores. You can be sure I'll be watching out for your budget, too, to make sure you also get the best buys.

Some of the worst choices include leafy green vegetables such as spinach and collards. Spinach's spongy leaves were saturated with 345 chemical pesticide residues in 44 samples, according to the FDA Total Diet Study that analyzed foods purchased from supermarkets throughout the nation.[14] Same for collards, a down-home, soul-food favorite of just about anybody else who loves Southern cuisine—there were 315 pesticide and industrial chemical residues in 44 samples.

Yet, these days, organically grown leafy greens are about the same price. Just get organic. It's that simple.

Among fruits, red apples were the worst with more than 340 chemical residues, followed by strawberries (321), peaches (293), raisins (269), and cherries (229) in 44 samples of each. Conventionally grown blueberries, raspberries, and blackberries have a similar toxic profile.

Fruit jams and jellies, all flavors, were contaminated with the OP pesticides and a newer chemical, azoxystrobin, a fungicide known to kill embryonic brain cells with profound gender effects in zebra fish, causing fewer males to be born, changing the shape and size of their gonads, and disrupting sex hormone production, leading to more intersex babies.[15] You don't need to feed your kids these chemicals. Buy organic jams and jelly. They come in all flavors and are the same price.

The fact is that competitively priced organic alternatives are available for these foods, too. Chains and shopping websites like Aldi, Amazon, Costco, Instacart, Kroger, Walmart, and Trader Joe's offer organically grown and sourced fruits and veggies, as well as prepared foods, at some of the lowest prices throughout the United States.

All of these outlets and other sources making organics accessible to far more people than ever before is a good thing—as long as standards are maintained.

Finally, if organic choices aren't available or cost too much, the safest conventionally grown veggies and fruits include these clean fifteen: asparagus, avocados, beets, baby carrots, spinach, and kale, cauliflower, corn, eggplant, garlic, green onions, honeydew, kiwi, mangoes, and watermelon.

## Safe and Unsafe Veggies

🛒 = Safe, none, or least risk from chemical toxins

🛒 = Dangerous, contains significant amounts of chemical toxins

All foods are conventionally grown unless otherwise noted

| Food | Reproductive and Developmental Toxicity | Cancer |
|---|---|---|
| Asparagus, fresh/frozen, boiled | 🛒 | 🛒 |
| Asparagus, fresh/frozen, boiled, organic | 🛒 | 🛒 |
| Beets, canned* | 🛒 | 🛒 |
| Beets, fresh | 🛒 | 🛒 |
| Beets, fresh, organic | 🛒 | 🛒 |
| Black beans | 🛒 | 🛒 |
| Black beans, organic | 🛒 | 🛒 |

| Food | Reproductive and Developmental Toxicity | Cancer |
|---|---|---|
| Bok choi | (filled cart) | (filled cart) |
| Bok choi, organic | (cart) | (cart) |
| Broccoli, fresh/frozen, boiled | (filled cart) | (filled cart) |
| Broccoli, organic | (cart) | (cart) |
| Cabbage, fresh, boiled | (cart) | (cart) |
| Cabbage, fresh, organic | (cart) | (cart) |
| Carrot, baby, raw | (cart) | (cart) |
| Carrot, baby, raw, organic | (cart) | (cart) |
| Carrot, fresh, peeled, boiled | (filled cart) | (filled cart) |
| Carrot, organic | (cart) | (cart) |
| Cauliflower, fresh/frozen, boiled | (cart) | (cart) |
| Cauliflower, organic | (cart) | (cart) |
| Celery, raw | (filled cart) | (filled cart) |
| Celery, raw, organic | (filled cart) | (filled cart) |
| Chayote | (cart) | (cart) |
| Chayote, organic | (cart) | (cart) |
| Chinese cabbage | (cart) | (cart) |
| Chinese cabbage, organic | (cart) | (cart) |
| Chinese radish/daikon | (filled cart) | (filled cart) |

*(Continued on next page)*

| Food | Reproductive and Developmental Toxicity | Cancer |
|---|---|---|
| Coleslaw with dressing, homemade | 🛒 | 🛒 |
| Collards, fresh/frozen, boiled | ⬤ | ⬤ |
| Collards, fresh/frozen, boiled, organic | 🛒 | 🛒 |
| Corn, canned* | 🛒 | 🛒 |
| Corn, canned, organic* | 🛒 | 🛒 |
| Corn, cream style, canned* | 🛒 | 🛒 |
| Corn, cream style, canned, organic* | 🛒 | 🛒 |
| Corn, sweet, fresh/frozen, boiled | 🛒 | 🛒 |
| Corn, sweet, fresh/frozen, boiled, organic | 🛒 | 🛒 |
| Cucumbers, peeled, raw | ⬤ | ⬤ |
| Cucumbers, raw, organic | 🛒 | 🛒 |
| Eggplant | 🛒 | 🛒 |
| Eggplant, organic | 🛒 | 🛒 |
| Fennel | ⬤ | ⬤ |
| Fennel, organic | 🛒 | 🛒 |
| Garbanzo beans | 🛒 | 🛒 |
| Garbanzo beans, organic | 🛒 | 🛒 |
| Garlic | 🛒 | 🛒 |
| Garlic, organic | 🛒 | 🛒 |

| Food | Reproductive and Developmental Toxicity | Cancer |
| --- | :---: | :---: |
| Ginger root | ● | ● |
| Ginger root, organic | ○ | ○ |
| Green beans, fresh/frozen, boiled | ● | ● |
| Green beans, fresh/frozen, boiled, organic | ● | ● |
| Green onions | ● | ● |
| Green onions, organic | ○ | ○ |
| Green string beans | ● | ● |
| Green string beans, organic | ○ | ○ |
| Jicama | ○ | ○ |
| Jicama, organic | ○ | ○ |
| Kale** | ● | ● |
| Kale, organic** | ● | ● |
| Kidney beans, dry, boiled | ○ | ○ |
| Lettuce, Iceberg, raw | ● | ● |
| Lettuce, Iceberg, raw, organic | ○ | ○ |
| Lettuce, leaf, raw | ● | ● |
| Lettuce, leaf, raw, organic | ○ | ○ |
| Lima beans, immature, frozen, boiled | ● | ● |
| Mint, spice | ○ | ○ |

*(Continued on next page)*

11

| Food | Reproductive and Developmental Toxicity | Cancer |
|------|:---:|:---:|
| Mixed vegetables, fresh/frozen, boiled | 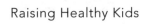 | ● |
| Mixed vegetables, fresh/frozen, boiled, organic | 🛒 | 🛒 |
| Mushrooms | ● | ● |
| Mushrooms, organic | 🛒 | 🛒 |
| Mustard greens | ● | ● |
| Mustard greens, organic | 🛒 | 🛒 |
| Okra, fresh/frozen, boiled | 🛒 | 🛒 |
| Okra, fresh/frozen, boiled, organic | 🛒 | 🛒 |
| Onion, green, raw | 🛒 | 🛒 |
| Onion, green, raw, organic | 🛒 | 🛒 |
| Onion, mature, raw | 🛒 | 🛒 |
| Onion, mature, raw, organic | 🛒 | 🛒 |
| Peas, green, frozen boiled | 🛒 | 🛒 |
| Peas, mature, dry, boiled | 🛒 | 🛒 |
| Peas, snow (sugar), organic | 🛒 | 🛒 |
| Pepper, chili | ● | ● |
| Pepper, chili, organic | 🛒 | 🛒 |
| Pepper, sweet, green, raw | ● | ● |
| Pepper, sweet, green, red, raw, organic | 🛒 | 🛒 |

| Food | Reproductive and Developmental Toxicity | Cancer |
|---|---|---|
| Potato, boiled (without peel) | ○ | ○ |
| Potato, mashed, prepared from fresh | ○ | ○ |
| Potato (with peel) | ● | ● |
| Potato (with peel), organic | ○ | ○ |
| Radish tops | ● | ● |
| Radish, raw | ● | ● |
| Radish tops, organic | ○ | ○ |
| Radish, raw, organic | ○ | ○ |
| Refried beans, canned* | ○ | ○ |
| Spinach, fresh/frozen, boiled | ● | ● |
| Spinach, organic* | ● | ● |
| Squash, winter (Hubbard/acorn), fresh/frozen, boiled | ● | ● |
| Squash, winter, organic | ○ | ○ |
| Squash, summer | ● | ● |
| Squash, summer, organic | ○ | ○ |
| Sweet potato | ○ | ○ |
| Sweet potato, organic | ○ | ○ |
| Swiss chard, organic | ● | ● |
| Tomatillo | ● | ● |

*(Continued on next page)*

| Food | Reproductive and Developmental Toxicity | Cancer |
|---|:---:|:---:|
| Tomato sauce, plain bottled |  |  |
| Tomato, raw |  |  |
| Tomato, organic |  |  |
| Turmeric, organic |  |  |
| Turnip, fresh/ frozen, boiled |  |  |
| Watermelon |  |  |
| Watermelon, organic |  |  |
| White beans, dry, boiled |  |  |
| Yam |  |  |
| Yam, organic |  |  |

\* Choose canned vegetables and beans from brands stating their products are free from the reproductive toxin bisphenol-A (BPA) and other bisphenol compounds. The BPAs are found in the cans' inner linings. They migrate into foods.

\*\* Spinach and kale are heavy metal accumulators. The amounts are high enough to warrant their exclusion from the diet of pregnant or nursing women and consumption of no more than once weekly for the rest of the population. Prefer baby spinach and kale, which will be much lower in heavy metals and toxic pesticides.

# Safe and Unsafe Fruits

🛒 = Safe, none, or least risk from chemical toxins

🛒 = Dangerous, contains significant amounts of chemical toxins

All foods are conventionally grown unless otherwise noted

| Food | Reproductive and Developmental Toxicity | Cancer |
|---|---|---|
| Apple (red), raw (with peel) | 🛒 | 🛒 |
| Apple (red), raw (with peel), organic | 🛒 | 🛒 |
| Applesauce, bottled | 🛒 | 🛒 |
| Applesauce, bottled, organic | 🛒 | 🛒 |
| Apricot, raw | 🛒 | 🛒 |
| Apricot, raw, organic | 🛒 | 🛒 |
| Apricots, canned in heavy/light syrup* | 🛒 | 🛒 |
| Asian pear | 🛒 | 🛒 |
| Asian pear, organic | 🛒 | 🛒 |
| Avocado, raw | 🛒 | 🛒 |
| Avocado, raw, organic | 🛒 | 🛒 |
| Banana, raw | 🛒 | 🛒 |
| Banana, organic | 🛒 | 🛒 |
| Blackberry | 🛒 | 🛒 |
| Blackberry, organic | 🛒 | 🛒 |
| Blueberry | 🛒 | 🛒 |
| Blueberry, organic | 🛒 | 🛒 |

*(Continued on next page)*

| Food | Reproductive and Developmental Toxicity | Cancer |
|---|---|---|
| Cantaloupe, raw/frozen | ● | ● |
| Cantaloupe, raw/frozen, organic | 🛒 | 🛒 |
| Cherries, sweet, raw | ● | ● |
| Cherries, sweet, raw, organic | 🛒 | 🛒 |
| Dragon fruit (pitaya) | ● | ● |
| Dragon fruit (pitaya), organic | 🛒 | 🛒 |
| Fig | ● | ● |
| Fig, organic | 🛒 | 🛒 |
| Fruit cocktail, canned in light syrup* | ● | ● |
| Fruit cocktail, canned in light syrup, organic* | 🛒 | 🛒 |
| Grapefruit, raw | ● | ● |
| Grapefruit, raw, organic | 🛒 | 🛒 |
| Grapes (red/green), raw | ● | ● |
| Grapes (red/green), raw, organic | 🛒 | 🛒 |
| Guava | ● | ● |
| Guava, organic | 🛒 | 🛒 |
| Honeydew melon | 🛒 | 🛒 |
| Honeydew melon, organic | 🛒 | 🛒 |
| Jam and jelly | ● | ● |
| Jam and jelly, organic | 🛒 | 🛒 |

| Food | Reproductive and Developmental Toxicity | Cancer |
|---|:---:|:---:|
| Kiwi fruit, raw | 🛒 | 🛒 |
| Kiwi fruit, raw, organic | 🛒 | 🛒 |
| Lemon, raw | 🛒 | 🛒 |
| Lemon, raw, organic | 🛒 | 🛒 |
| Lime, raw | ● | ● |
| Lime, raw, organic | 🛒 | 🛒 |
| Mango, raw | 🛒 | 🛒 |
| Mango, organic | 🛒 | 🛒 |
| Nectarines, raw | ● | ● |
| Nectarines, raw, organic | 🛒 | 🛒 |
| Orange (navel/Valencia) raw | ● | ● |
| Orange, raw, organic | 🛒 | 🛒 |
| Papaya, raw | ● | ● |
| Papaya, raw, organic | 🛒 | 🛒 |
| Peach, canned in light/medium syrup* | ● | ● |
| Peach, canned in light/medium syrup, organic* | 🛒 | 🛒 |
| Peach, raw/frozen | ● | ● |
| Peach, raw/frozen, organic | 🛒 | 🛒 |
| Pear, canned in light syrup* | 🛒 | 🛒 |

*(Continued on next page)*

| Food | Reproductive and Developmental Toxicity | Cancer |
|---|---|---|
| Pear, raw (w/ peel) | 🛒 | 🛒 |
| Pear, raw (w/ peel), organic | 🛒 | 🛒 |
| Pineapple, raw | 🛒 | 🛒 |
| Pineapple, raw, organic | 🛒 | 🛒 |
| Pineapple, canned in juice* | 🛒 | 🛒 |
| Plums, purple, raw | 🛒 | 🛒 |
| Plums, purple, raw, organic | 🛒 | 🛒 |
| Pomegranate | 🛒 | 🛒 |
| Pomegranate, organic | 🛒 | 🛒 |
| Prickly pear cactus | 🛒 | 🛒 |
| Prickly pear cactus, organic | 🛒 | 🛒 |
| Prunes, dried, uncooked | 🛒 | 🛒 |
| Prunes, dried, uncooked, organic | 🛒 | 🛒 |
| Raisins | 🛒 | 🛒 |
| Raisins, organic | 🛒 | 🛒 |
| Raspberry, raw | 🛒 | 🛒 |
| Raspberry, raw, organic | 🛒 | 🛒 |
| Strawberries, raw/frozen | 🛒 | 🛒 |
| Strawberries, raw/frozen, organic | 🛒 | 🛒 |

| Food | Reproductive and Developmental Toxicity | Cancer |
|---|---|---|
| Tangelo, raw | 🛒 | 🛒 |
| Tangelo, raw, organic | 🛒 | 🛒 |
| Tangerine, raw | 🛒 | 🛒 |
| Tangerine, raw, organic | 🛒 | 🛒 |
| Watermelon, raw/frozen | 🛒 | 🛒 |
| Watermelon, raw/frozen, organic | 🛒 | 🛒 |

\* Choose canned fruits from brands stating their products are free from BPA and other bisphenol compounds.

## Organic Juice, Please

Conventionally sourced apple juice had 85 chemical toxins (including many OP pesticides) in 44 samples. Orange and grapefruit juices had 108 and 57 toxic residues, respectively. Grape, cranberry, tomato, prune, and fruit juices were contaminated with OPs. Pineapple juice was the least contaminated. Organic apple, grape, orange, and fruit juices are similarly priced to conventionally sourced products. Choose these instead.

### Safe and Unsafe Fruit and Vegetable Juices*

🛒 = Safe, none, or least risk from chemical toxins
🛒 = Dangerous, contains significant amounts of chemical toxins
All foods are conventionally grown unless otherwise noted

| Food | Reproductive and Developmental Toxicity | Cancer |
|---|---|---|
| Apple, bottled | 🛒 | 🛒 |
| Apple, organic | 🛒 | 🛒 |
| Coconut | 🛒 | 🛒 |

*(Continued on next page)*

| Food | Reproductive and Developmental Toxicity | Cancer |
|---|---|---|
| Coconut, organic | 🛒 | 🛒 |
| Cranberry | ⬤🛒 | ⬤🛒 |
| Cranberry, organic | 🛒 | 🛒 |
| Grape, frozen concentrate, reconstituted | ⬤🛒 | ⬤🛒 |
| Grape, organic | 🛒 | 🛒 |
| Grapefruit, frozen, concentrated, reconstituted | ⬤🛒 | ⬤🛒 |
| Grapefruit, organic | 🛒 | 🛒 |
| Orange, frozen concentrate, reconstituted | ⬤🛒 | ⬤🛒 |
| Orange frozen concentrate, reconstituted, organic | 🛒 | 🛒 |
| Pineapple | 🛒 | 🛒 |
| Pineapple, organic | 🛒 | 🛒 |
| Prune | ⬤🛒 | ⬤🛒 |
| Prune, organic | 🛒 | 🛒 |
| Tomato | 🛒 | 🛒 |
| Tomato, organic | 🛒 | 🛒 |

\* Choose canned juices from brands stating their products are free from BPA and other bisphenol compounds.

## Who Doesn't Love a Frozen Dessert?

Buy those two- and three-pound bags of frozen organic veggies and fruits. They're less expensive, keep longer, are more nutritious, and frozen organic strawberries or blueberries make a super tasty kids' dessert when sprinkled over a bowl of nonfat yogurt.

## *Shop the Seasons*

Following the seasons eliminates the need for imports and resulting transportation-related greenhouse gas emissions, which is good for your pocketbook and our planet.

In the winter, I look for organically grown avocados, broccoli, cabbage, collards, onions, spinach, squash, and yams. Citrus comes into its own during the winter with low prices for organic grapefruit, mandarins, oranges, and tangerines. Look for some of our more elusive and prized fruits too: kiwis, pears, persimmons, raspberries, and strawberries.

Spring brings on a colorful palette of asparagus, carrots, fava beans, mushrooms, radishes, and sugar snap peas. I'm thinking stir fries with broccoli florets, baby carrots, and a low-toxin protein like chicken, tofu, or shrimp. Organic apricots, honeydew melons, pineapple, and blackberries are plentiful on store shelves.

Summer is time for corn, cucumbers, eggplant, garlic, green beans, all colors of peppers, and zucchini. It's definitely the season to grill your favorite organic veggies and low-toxin proteins on metal skewers over the barbecue. Summer fruits add much-needed antioxidants to your child's diet, and nothing beats organic blueberries, cherries, peaches, plums, and watermelon for a sweet and healthy treat.

Fall veggies—beets, cauliflower, celery, chives, green beans, baby kale and spinach, pumpkins, and romaine lettuce—reach the markets from late August to November. Fall is also a time of plenty and lower prices for apples, bananas, cranberries, figs, mangoes, and pomegranates.

Share with your kids how some veggies and fruits are plentiful during different times of the year. Be colorful with your presentations. Every season has its colors.

## *Wash, Pare, and Preserve*

With all leafy greens, thoroughly washing them with a mild veggie soap can remove some of the accumulated cadmium, lead, and pesticides.[16, 17] This is especially important for spinach, kale, collards, and lettuce whose leaves are sponges for pesticides, heavy metals, or both. (In Chapter 11, I'll share with you how to filter your tap water to make sure you don't re-contaminate your foods when washing them.)

Some pesticides in conventionally sourced foods can be removed by paring or removing the skin. Potatoes are sprayed with post-harvest pesticides to prevent sprouting. Removing their skin reduces exposure to them. Paring carrots, cucumbers, and other fruits and veggies can also help eliminate some surface poisons.

Organics require extra care to preserve their shelf life. Take these simple steps:

- Wrap moisture-absorbing paper towels around celery, lettuce, other leafy greens, and soft-skinned items to keep them dry and extend their shelf life in the refrigerator.
- Slip a paper towel into your packaged greens to give them several days of added life.
- Onions, potatoes, and other root crops can be stored in a light-blocking bag in a cool pantry.
- Keep corn in the husk and in the fridge until you're ready to cook it.

On the other hand, take it from me, organic oranges, mandarins, and tangerines can last for months and still taste sweet.

Two years into the pandemic, I returned to Salinas. I parked in front of the Lagunita School with its steeple roof. The school is basically for farmworkers' kids and surrounded by agricultural fields. I gazed past the playground that abutted the rolling hills of leafy green strawberries growing there now with diamond-sparkling plastic spread over the verdant loam. Flat-bed trucks, Ford and Dodge pickups, some with crew cabs, tractors, and small cars—none new, all dented—lined the distant roads. I spotted a sign staked into the ground by the road with the first two lines of black lettering and rest in red:

**Alejandro Ramirez**
**Organic Strawberries**
***No Se Permiten Pesticidas***
**No Pesticides Permitted**

A few miles away, I drove down a quiet broad road, past a gray-white house that rose in the middle of a large patchy grass lawn with eucalyptus, palm, and oak trees, that ran up to a tattered, uneven picket fence. A silvery, shiny windmill towered over the motionless tree limbs.

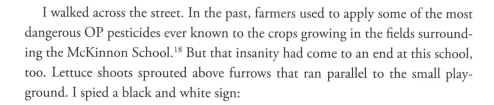

I walked across the street. In the past, farmers used to apply some of the most dangerous OP pesticides ever known to the crops growing in the fields surrounding the McKinnon School.[18] But that insanity had come to an end at this school, too. Lettuce shoots sprouted above furrows that ran parallel to the small playground. I spied a black and white sign:

**Organic Farm**
**Do Not Spray**
***Rancho Organico***
***No Aplicar Pesticidas***

I saw kids happily running out of their classrooms to the play area. They were safe now.

I called Oscar.

"How did this happen?" I said, my voice filled with excitement.

"It's thanks to shoppers like you who're buying those organic strawberries," Oscar said. "You're making the difference. I mean, we're working with local officials all of the time, but it's the consumer demand that's making it happen."

A lot more still needs to be done, he reminded me as we said goodbye. "But this is real progress and means a lot to these kids' lives."

I drove home that night with a sense of being part of something larger, moving our nation's historic arc toward greater justice for all. But would the kids at the schools I'd seen earlier ever connect their improved health today to what local activists like Oscar Ramos did for them yesterday—or have been doing their entire lives? I wondered. Probably not, I suspected. Yet, that didn't daunt Oscar or me one bit. I thought what I witnessed at the schools with my own two eyes was a real-life miracle. Discovering what I had—that confirmed an act of faith. Buying all of those organic strawberries really did make a difference in people's lives.

I lived three hundred miles south of Salinas. But Oscar, Daisy, their families, and the many other teachers, parents, researchers, and youths who shared their stories led me to realize how close we really are to each other. I just didn't know how much we had been going through together.

It doesn't cost much more to buy organic foods for your own kids. And when you do, it's like taking care of everyone and everywhere all at once.

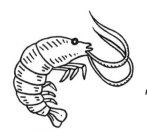

# Chapter 2

# The Catch

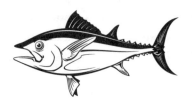

I first learned of the toxins in sport fish caught from the waters of the Santa Monica Bay when I was covering environmental issues in the mid-1980s as an investigative reporter at *L.A. Weekly*. Initially, reporters focused their attention on dolphins whose carcasses, highly contaminated with chemical toxins, had washed up on the local beaches. But I knew the poisoning didn't stop there.

The paper's news editor asked me to do what I initially considered impossible: get thirty strangers who regularly consumed fish from the bay to give me their blood to measure the levels of their pesticides and industrial chemicals.

I put together a team that consisted of a physician (Gary Wikholm, a childhood friend) who was fluent in both Spanish and English, an analytical chemist, a marine biologist, and a pathologist, the last two of whom were affiliated with the University of Southern California.

We traveled that summer, armed with syringes, needles, test tubes, latex gloves, and consumption questionnaires, to the piers and sport fishing landings throughout Los Angeles County. Honestly, I don't know how we got done what we did. I know now you have to be crazy and desperate (in a good way). I mean, Wikholm was a full-fledged doctor, delivering babies in a white smock at Glendale Adventist, a Loma Linda University–affiliated medical center, after all. But here with us out on the piers, he had on khaki pants, Hawaiian shirt, and straw hat. He had a cocky attitude and Fu Manchu mustache. But everyone trusted him. After all, he handled those needles like a real professional.

Our marine biologist, John Ljubenkov, standing six foot seven, with long brown hair past his shoulders, could have passed for Neptune the sea god himself. He had a booming voice that could be heard one hundred feet away and naturally attracted people as he queried our participants to determine the frequency and amount of local seafood they consumed per month.

I made myself into an ambassador of sorts, approaching folks, introducing myself and the rest of the team, telling a prospective participant we were offering them a deal.

We needed around three dozen persons to give us their blood (for a statistically significant sampling) in exchange for free laboratory work valued at more than five hundred dollars, I explained.

I told them we would analyze their blood levels for two chemicals known as dichlorodiphenyltrichloroethane (DDT) and polychlorinated biphenyls (PCBs), both of which last for decades in the environment, build up in the fatty tissues of animals and humans, and are carcinogens and fetal toxins. A lot of folks wanted to know if they had high levels from eating the locally caught fish, thought it was a good deal, and volunteered.

First stop was the fog-shrouded, concrete-gray Venice Pier with its weathered, notched-wood railings lined by fishers dropping down their lines into the frothy swells, splashing against mussel-covered pilings.

"I eat fish here all the time," a Japanese American man told us when we asked him if we could sample his blood.

Freckles sprinkled over his face's parchment-thin skin. His hands were covered with sunspots. He positioned his rod in a notch in the wood rail.

"I was a postal worker," he said as he bared his arm for the doctor who tightened the elastic tourniquet.

The man's veins popped out, and the doctor slipped in his needle. Our volunteer spoke as his blood flowed into the syringe.

"I come here to fish every day. See."

His bucket was filled with stiffening, milky-white croakers floating belly up. Those were the worst fish with the most DDT. I didn't know what to say to him, so I said something innocuous and, in retrospect, insensitive.

"Do you still deliver the mail?" I asked.

"No, I have liver cancer," he replied casually and smiled. I still remember his crinkly brown eyes and kind smile. His wife stood nearby, tightlipped, watching her husband.

I watched his dark burgundy blood fill the vial.

At the end of our visit, we were nearby where the pier pilings drilled into the seashore, closer to the palm trees. We spotted an African American woman in a yellow sundress off to one side and approached her. The wind blew shining specks of sand past us; she was flipping freshly caught perch fillets on a small hibachi-style barbecue set on three spindly, silvery legs on a concrete slab. Her baby daughter, swathed in blankets, was snugly ensconced in a stroller with a canopy to shade her from the sun. Her husband stood a football field or two away by the sturdy pier pilings, casting his line into the white surf. He was fishing for barred surf perch, strolling down into the water, casting out, and waiting.

The little fishes were hungry, and he brought up a wriggling barred surf perch for his partner to grill. We said hello quickly, talked, and he went back to catch more.

"Nothing more sweet," she said, grilling them right there on the beach until their silvery skin and white flesh were crisp.

"I'd definitely like to know what's in my blood," she said, putting down the silver spatula, baring the underside of her arm. "I got my baby and kids. I want to know 'cause we come here all the time to fish and barbecue."

On another trip, this time to the South Bay, we went to Redondo Beach. The captain of a sport-fishing party boat operating out of King Harbor boldly offered up her arm to draw blood.

"We got nothing to fear," she said with a New England accent and confidence that was almost dismissive. Wikholm slipped his needle into her arm above a dragon tattoo. The captain told the doctor she suffered hypertension and gave him her most recent readings while blood filled the syringe.

"The fish are pure," said the cook as he turned from the grill to face us. He wore a sleeveless undershirt and chef's white apron over it. He had a smooth hairless face and pug nose and demanded, "Take my blood too."

"The problem's the beef," he went on as the doctor slipped a needle into his vein. "It's why I don't eat beef burgers. I'll eat fish burgers but no beef, you got me? No beef. Or lettuce. It's the lettuce, I bet. They spray all sorts of stuff on lettuce. You don't know how bad it is."

The cook truly believed the seafood in their very own bay was safe, and I knew no matter what the results were, we would never convince him he was being poisoned by his fish burgers. But if he was, he had already concocted a rationale to protect his interests.

"You don't think it's the DDT in the lettuce?" the cook called.

We left with half a dozen vials of blood including from some of the men and women we fished with earlier.

A few weeks later, we knew one of the reasons the captain had high blood pressure. She had among the study's highest concentrations of DDT and PCBs. Both cause hypertension.[1, 2] Her cook's blood also harbored high amounts of both.

The blood of the Japanese American man was loaded too.

Nobody can say for sure whether the DDT was the cause of his liver cancer. But the high levels didn't help. And we do know DDT causes liver cancers.

We visited the mother we had met at her home in Bellflower. It had a lawn and tattered picket fence and was across the road that ran alongside the freeway. Wikholm and I sat together on the couch. She sat in a chair with a high back, holding her baby, in her cozy, crowded living room with its colonial furniture and fake ivory fireplace. The room looked out on a concrete corridor across the street, covered with ivy, built to reduce the passing cars' drone.

"You had one hundred forty parts per billion of the pesticide in your blood," said Wikholm, leaning forward earnestly.

"Is that a lot?" she said softly.

He nodded.

"Most people have a few parts per billion," he said.

"It in her too?" she asked, holding her baby close.

"Well, it's in your breast milk . . ." Wikholm's voice trailed off.

"Why they let that in me?"

She looked at me and then down at her baby who was quiet. We heard the swoosh of the speeding cars barreling down the freeway.

"It was covered up for a long time—people around here were getting poisoned," I said. "We're going to publish what happened in the *L.A. Weekly*, and you're going to help us make a difference. Our state water resources board allowed Montrose, the chemical company, to barge thousands of tons of DDT waste sludge from its plant into the Catalina Channel and dump it in barrels they hacked open to sink into the sea. They thought it would all go away and disappear. Dilute into nothing. Instead, it's concentrating in the fish and the people who eat them." I struggled to find the words. "It's so stupid . . . so shortsighted . . . Montrose wasn't thinking of us. They had a mess and just wanted to dump it someplace. They didn't care and apparently neither did the folks on the water board who gave them their permission."

"Now they let me get it in my child. What you and me gonna do?" she said, looking back at Wikholm.

"That's why we're trying to get people to pay attention to this issue," he said.

"My baby gonna be okay?" she asked, plaintively.

"She will be," the doctor said. "But you have to cut down on eating the fish from the bay, okay?"

She nodded, and we walked out, feeling awful, just terrible at having to bear such horrible news. There was no support network for any of our victims. None. No one was going to help them. Ever. They were invisible.

"It isn't just the people at the piers getting poisoned," Wikholm said when we got in my car. It was dark now, and we could hear the whirring traffic. Finding out there were so many people being poisoned was a true life-changing experience for all of us who were conducting the study. But, for me, it was personal. I had my blood analyzed too. The lab found high amounts of DDT in my blood. I was one of the poisoned.

I had fished all of my life and, before becoming an investigative reporter at *L.A. Weekly*, worked in San Pedro on a purse-seine fishing boat called *Janie II* netting mackerel for the cannery, living on locally caught halibut, sea bass, bonito, opaleye, calico bass, and the occasional sea urchins we brought in with our catch. I cannot adequately describe to you the sense of betrayal I felt when I got my results.

Looking back on events now, it all makes sense in a horrible way. Nobody was looking out for me.

I came to realize if I continued to eat poisoned local seafood, my blood pollution concentrations could only worsen.

Wikholm was no doubt one of the poisoned, too. After all, he and I had fished perch and flounder in the bay from childhood when we could walk from our homes to the big, broad whales' mouth of an estuary fed by the Ballona Creek, emptying into the sea where there is now a marina. He knew he was poisoned. He had to know. He took everyone else's blood, but he couldn't do his own, of course, he said, because he was conducting the study. But I don't think he wanted to know. All he cared about were his patients whom he saw in the faces of that mother and child whose home we just left. A lot of mothers with young kids who came to him ate locally caught seafood. It was less expensive and always fresh.

"Thousands of pounds of mackerel, bonito, barracuda, black cod, white croakers, halibut, and sea bass are being caught every night by the commercial fishing boats and sold directly into the seafood markets the next day throughout Los Angeles and Orange County," he said. "Choose the wrong species and you're going to accumulate poisons. This is a catastrophe." We looked at each other and laughed as if we were going to the gallows.

As it turned out, our investigation, published in *L.A. Weekly* and, subsequently, *Environmental Toxicology and Chemistry*, led to a joint state and federal hearing before the congressional Health and Environment Subcommittee, chaired by Representative Henry Waxman.[3] Santa Monica Bay was declared a Federal Superfund site, which provided funding for its cleanup, following our testimony.[4] The nonprofit group Heal the Bay was formed by my late friend Dorothy Green to watch over the cleanup. I also reported that Montrose chemical company, manufacturing DDT in south Los Angeles, was responsible for this ecological disaster. The company barged its waste sludge into the Catalina Channel and dumped some two thousand tons into the deep blue waters where it became part of the ecosystem. The pesticide worked its way up into the high-level predatory fish the sport and commercial fishers caught. Those who consumed the seafood had DDT and PCB levels as much as ten times higher than people who did not eat local fish. Montrose was eventually part of a $73 million dollar settlement to help clean up the bay.[5]

The tragedy for our nation is that, despite clean water legislation that was passed in the early 1970s, the chemical contamination of our seafood is only worsening.

About half of consumers shop by availability and price, one research team found while studying New Jersey's seafood markets. This means shoppers are buying a lot of flounder, snapper, tuna, whiting, porgy, croaker, and bluefish from local waters with high amounts of pollutants and no warnings.[6]

Even today, most people don't have the faintest idea about the chemical load of their fish and shellfish choices.

Yet, the seafood choices persons of reproductive age or who are pregnant make are being made for two and, in that way, even more significant.

The time to start finding safe seafood is now. The toxic chemicals found in seafood are long-lasting and accumulate in the blood and fatty tissues. It takes months and consistent low-toxin shopping habits to lower your levels. The good news is that being more careful with your seafood choices can go a long way toward reducing the amount of chemical toxins in your body. This allows you to make sure your kids never experience what I did when no one told me about the fish that were poisoned.

## The Catch—A Family Protection Plan

Some seafood choices should be avoided by everybody who cares about their health. These seafood choices with the highest chemical concentrations aren't safe for anybody, much less the fetus or kids.

Before you get depressed if I call out one of your favorites for having too much contamination, just remember we have plenty of safe seafood choices. I'll share these as well.

### *Avoid*

**European (Scottish and Norwegian) and Faroe Islands salmon**, farmed or wild, have high PCB levels.[7, 8]

**Yellowfin tuna, caught from the northeast Atlantic, Gulf of Mexico, and waters close to industrialized shores**, have high amounts of mercury and DDT.[9, 10]

**Albacore** (shiro maguro when ordering sushi), known as white tuna when canned, typically contains three times more mercury than chunk light and should be avoided during pregnancy and by infants and children.

Sadly for fans of *Wicked Tuna*, the popular National Geographic series, **bluefin landed from the waters of the northeast Atlantic or Mediterranean** are PCB, DDT, and mercury sinks. Too bad because their fatty flesh makes for some of the best sushi.

**Gefilte fish**, a Jewish food enjoyed on the Sabbath, **prepared from northern pike, walleye, and carp**, is tainted with DDT and highly toxic forever chemicals called per- and polyfluoroalkyl substances (PFAS) that cause cancer, kidney disease, and feminize the male anatomy.[11] The HLF tested four leading brands including Manischewitz, Yehuda, Rokeach, and Benz's; all were PFAS contaminated.

**Catfish**, a traditional Asian and Southern food, whether river-caught or farm-raised, is a cause of PCB accumulation, especially among African Americans.[12]

**Carp**, a mainstay of some Asian cultures, whether wild or farmed, is way too high in DDT, PCBs, and PFAS.[13]

**Snakehead fish**, popular in Asian cuisine, are loaded with PCBs.[14]

**King and Spanish mackerel**, used in Vietnamese and Russian dishes, are high in mercury and DDT.

**Herring from the waters of the Northeastern US or Baltic** usually contain PCBs.

**Striped, smallmouth, and largemouth bass, perch, sunfish, bream, crappie, chub, lake trout, and virtually all other freshwater species from anywhere in the US** are likely to be high in pesticides, mercury, PCBs, PFAS, and other industrial chemicals.[15]

**Sturgeon from America's inland waters such as the Columbia and Missouri rivers** are contaminated with pesticides so high they are suffering from blurred sexual organs and chemically induced reproductive difficulties.[16, 17] **Sturgeon roe from European fish** is consumed as caviar but also tainted.[18]

**All canned clam, mussel, and oyster products from China** should be avoided. These are all high in lead and cadmium and, consumed even once, pose a dire reproductive hazard to the fetus. More recently, PFAS are also being detected in their edible portions.[19]

**Shun sea-ranched abalone from China.** Sea-ranching involves clearing large areas of ocean bottom as though they are pastures, altering the natural habitat, and creating ecological mayhem. Just assume, unless otherwise stated, abalone from China will have been raised in this manner.

Avoid **mahi-mahi (dolphinfish) caught using longlines**. Be sure your seller specifies the method of catch; otherwise, avoid.

## Hooray, Your Safest Choices!

America and Europe's most popular seafood choice, **shrimp** (called ebi in sushi), if taken from the wild, is safe during pregnancy and for kids as well as adults. Shrimp is a valuable source of calcium, protein, heart-healthy omega-3 fatty acids, and iodine.

Thankfully, we salmon lovers have our **wild sockeye** (called sake in sushi) from Chile and Alaska, which are as pure as the seven seas. [20] [21] Wild or farm-raised salmon (called suzuki as sashimi) from Chile and Washington are safe.

Thank the sea gods for the fast-swimming **skipjack**. It's the smallest of all tuna, the most prolific species, and definitely the number-one safe choice for kids. Chunk light tuna made from skipjack is not only the least expensive kind but has the lowest amounts of mercury and toxic pesticide residues. Skipjack populations are stable. Make tuna salad for the kids with organic mayonnaise, celery, and relish on sandwich bread for a healthy lunch.

If you do buy **yellowfin tuna**, those from the Northern and Southern Pacific, South Atlantic, and Indian oceans are most free from pollution. Wild Planet offers sustainably caught yellowfin from these waters. Crown Prince Natural sources their tuna from the waters of Thailand. Safe Catch has instituted complete tracing for its tuna, which are taken from the Western Central Pacific. Whole Foods Market sells pole- and line-caught yellowfin from the Pacific Northwest and Maldives, regions farther from relevant pollution sources.

**Pacific cod, pollock, haddock, and sole** from Alaska are used for fish sticks. Their levels of contaminants are low, too. But here's the catch: when battered, as with fish sticks, their crust is rife with organophosphate (OP) pesticides that are toxic to kids' nervous systems. On the other hand, organic batters are available if you want to make your own. Some of my favorites include: Edward & Sons Organic Panko Breadcrumbs, O Organics, and Simple Truth. You can also grill, broil, or bake with herbs as a low-toxin seafood meal.

I gave you the bad news for gefilte fish. Fortunately, there's good news, too, for fans of the homemade variety. Joan Nathan, writing in *The New York Times* that she's never been a big fan of canned and bottled varieties, reminds us that "a mix of fatty fish, like salmon, striped bass or even whitefish, goes well with trout or the traditional pike, carp or mullet. You could substitute any fish as long as it has fins and scales, according to Jewish dietary laws."[22]

For those who make their own gefilte fish, plenty of much safer choices, including sockeye salmon, pollock, cod, haddock, and tilapia, are available. With the right seasonings, they will capture the same iconic gefilte fish flavor. I recommend starting with the easily prepared recipe for "Salmon and Cod Gefilte Fish" at Marthastewart.com.

**Pacific or Alaskan flounder** (called hirami in sushi) is preferred over the Northeastern Atlantic species.

**Red drum**, a staple of Louisiana's world-famous Cajun seafood, is low in chemical toxins.

**Alaskan king, snow, stone, blue, Dungeness, and southern tanner crabs** (called kani in sushi) are safe.

**Lobster** including the spiny West Coast variety (called ise-ebi in sushi), except for the portion called the tomalley (the soft, green substance found in its body cavity), is permissible.[23]

**Abalone** (called awabi in sushi), a staple of Asian cuisine that is wild-harvested or farmed using barrels and enclosed containers, is safe.

**Octopus** (called tako in sushi) is safe to consume.

So are **squid and sea urchin** (called iki and uni, respectively, in sushi).

**Surimi** (used in California rolls) is safe.

**Pacific halibut** (called hoshigarei in sushi) has low levels of PCBs. It's the safest halibut but limit to once a month.

**Tilapia** (called izumidai in sushi), with its sweet mild flavor, is one of my kids' favorites. It's an economic, safe choice.[24]

**Trout** caught from high mountain lakes and streams and rivers before they flow into the bottom and lowlands of the nation are safe. Farm-raised trout is also safe.

When caught by pole or trolling, **mahi-mahi** and **Pacific yellowtail** are both safe enough to enjoy once or twice a month during pregnancy and for persons of childbearing age.

## Four Questions Savvy Seafood Shoppers Need to Ask

When you find yourself dining out or shopping for seafood, be sure to ask these questions to make a safe choice:

1. **Is it small or big?** Smaller fish—such as anchovies, sardines, sand dabs, and skipjack—generally contain less contaminants than larger species like bluefin tuna, swordfish, and shark.
2. **Is my catch farmed or wild?** In some cases, wild catch is preferred as with wild-caught Alaskan sockeye salmon.[25] However, I'd pass on both farm-raised or wild-caught carp, catfish, and European salmon.

3. **Where is my catch from?** Seafood shoppers often can't get the information they need from their local supermarket fish monger (although some supermarkets and online sites tend to be more informative). But Wild Planet, Safe Catch, and a few other brands do provide information about where and how their seafood is caught. Patronize seafood shops that know where their seafood comes from, so you can make an informed choice. Seafood from Alaska and South America, especially Chile and Peru, and the Central Pacific, consistently delivers the purest catch. Shellfish from Chile, the Oregon coast, and Prince Edward Island also tend to be the most pure. Also, pay attention to local fish advisories, available online, and provided by state environmental health departments. Seafoodwatch.org, a project of the Monterey Bay Aquarium, is an important information source for making sustainable choices.

4. **How is my seafood prepared and cooked?** Good news for those who grill or broil. Grilling and broiling, where the fat drips off the fish, are thought to be the most effective cooking methods for reducing levels. Frying could actually increase concentrations.[26] Removing the skin reduces concentrations by as much as 9 percent.[27] The combination of removing the skin and grilling is thought to be the best way to prepare seafood. Keep the grilling light to avoid charring with combustion byproducts that are toxic to children's cells.

## Safe and Unsafe Seafood

🛒 = Safe, none, or least risk from chemical toxins

⬤ = Dangerous, contains significant amounts of chemical toxins

| Food Item | Reproductive and Developmental Risk | Cancer Risk |
|---|---|---|
| Albacore tuna | Safe | Safe |
| Bluefin tuna | Dangerous | Dangerous |
| Bluefish | Dangerous | Dangerous |
| Bumble Bee Fancy Smoked Oysters (canned) | Dangerous | Dangerous |
| Carp | Dangerous | Dangerous |

| Food Item | Reproductive and Developmental Risk | Cancer Risk |
|---|:---:|:---:|
| Catfish (farmed) | ● | ● |
| Catfish (wild) | ● | ● |
| Caviar | ● | ● |
| Clams (baby, chopped) | ○ | ○ |
| Clams (Chile) | ○ | ○ |
| Clams (China) | ● | ● |
| Clams (Prince Edward Island) | ○ | ○ |
| Cod | ○ | ○ |
| Crab (Alaskan king, snow, stone, blue, dungeness, and southern tanner) | ○ | ○ |
| Crappie | ● | ● |
| Dover Sole | ○ | ○ |
| Flounder (Alaska) | ○ | ○ |
| Flounder (Northeastern US) | ● | ● |
| Halibut (Alaskan) | ○ | ○ |
| Hood Canal Oysters | ● | ● |
| Kumamoto Oysters | ○ | ○ |
| Lake trout | ● | ● |
| Mackerel (all species) | ● | ● |
| Mahi-mahi (longline) | ● | ● |
| Mahi-mahi (pole or trolling) | ○ | ○ |
| Manischewitz Gefilte Fish | ● | ● |
| Mussels (Chile) | ○ | ○ |
| Mussels (China) | ● | ● |

*(Continued on next page)*

| Food Item | Reproductive and Developmental Risk | Cancer Risk |
|---|:---:|:---:|
| Mussels (China, sold by M.W. Polar, Reese, Roland) | ● | ● |
| Mussels (Maine) | ● | ● |
| Mussels (Prince Edward Island) | ○ | ○ |
| Mussels (Spain) | ● | ● |
| Oysters (China, sold by Bumble Bee, California Girl, Chicken of the Sea, Crown Prince, Geisha, M.W. Polar, Reese, Roland) | ● | ● |
| Oysters (Oregon coast) | ○ | ○ |
| Pacific halibut | ○ | ○ |
| Pollock (Alaskan) | ○ | ○ |
| Salmon (farmed) | ● | ● |
| Salmon (wild chinook, coho, and sockeye) | ○ | ○ |
| Saltwater eel (China, Europe, Japan)[28] | ● | ● |
| Scallops (China, Philippines Spain) | ● | ● |
| Scallops (Mexico) | ○ | ○ |
| Shrimp (wild harvested) | ○ | ○ |
| Skipjack | ○ | ○ |
| Snapper (Gulf Coast) | ● | ● |
| Surimi | ○ | ○ |
| Sturgeon | ● | ● |
| Swordfish | ● | ● |
| Tilapia | ○ | ○ |
| Trout (alpine) | ○ | ○ |
| Trout (farm-raised) | ○ | ○ |

| Food Item | Reproductive and Developmental Risk | Cancer Risk |
|---|:---:|:---:|
| Yellowfin (Central Western Pacific) | 🛒 | 🛒 |
| Yellowfin (Gulf of Mexico, Northeastern US) | ⚫ | ⚫ |
| Yellowtail (Japan) | 🛒 | 🛒 |
| Yellowtail (Pacific Ocean)[29] | 🛒 | 🛒 |

Nearly one-third of Americans have eaten sushi in the last year.[30] Choose sushi bars that routinely serve sashimi-grade skipjack, the safe and most plentiful tuna, or yellowfin from the Central Pacific or Southern Atlantic. California rolls made with surimi are safe. Please note the seaweed that wraps the rice in sushi rolls binds heavy metals and radiation absorbed by your body from the environment and diet and helps eliminate them, aiding detoxification. Seaweed is also thought to inhibit breast as well as other cancers.[31] Seaweed's iodine content protects against radiation fallout.[32] Meanwhile, many safe sushi choices deliver heart-healthy omega-3 fatty acids.[33]

## Safe and Unsafe Sushi

| 🛒 = Safe, none, or least risk from chemical toxins |
|---|
| ⚫ = Dangerous, contains significant amounts of chemical toxins |

| Sushi | Reproductive and Developmental Risk | Cancer Risk |
|---|:---:|:---:|
| Aji (horse mackerel) | ⚫ | ⚫ |
| Anago (saltwater eel)[34] | ⚫ | ⚫ |
| Awabi (abalone) | 🛒 | 🛒 |
| Buri (adult yellowtail)[35] | ⚫ | ⚫ |
| Ebi (shrimp) | 🛒 | 🛒 |
| Gindara (sablefish) | ⚫ | ⚫ |

| Sushi | Reproductive and Developmental Risk | Cancer Risk |
|---|---|---|
| Hamachi (juvenile yellowtail) | ● | ● |
| Hamguri (clams) | ● | ● |
| Hirami (flounder, northeastern) | ● | ● |
| Hirami (flounder, Pacific or Alaskan) | ◦ | ◦ |
| Hoshigarei (Pacific halibut) | ◦ | ◦ |
| Hotate (scallops) | ● | ● |
| Iki (squid) | ◦ | ◦ |
| Ikura (salmon roe) | ● | ● |
| Ise-ebi (lobster except for the tomalley) | ◦ | ◦ |
| Iwana (arctic char) | ● | ● |
| Izumidai (tilapia) | ◦ | ◦ |
| Kajiki (swordfish) | ● | ● |
| Kaki (oysters) | ● | ● |
| Makizushi roll (spicy tuna, bluefin) | ● | ● |
| Makizushi roll (spicy tuna, skipjack) | ◦ | ◦ |
| Makizushi roll (spicy tuna, yellowfin) | ● | ● |
| Masago (smelt roe) | ● | ● |
| Masiju (trout) | ● | ● |
| Mirugai (giant clam) | ● | ● |

| Sushi | Reproductive and Developmental Risk | Cancer Risk |
|---|---|---|
| Muurugai (mussels) | 🛒 (filled) | 🛒 (filled) |
| Saba (mackerel) | 🛒 (filled) | 🛒 (filled) |
| Shiro maguro (albacore tuna) | 🛒 (outline) | 🛒 (outline) |
| Surimi (artificial crab) | 🛒 (outline) | 🛒 (outline) |
| Suzuki (sea bass) | 🛒 (filled) | 🛒 (filled) |
| Tako (octopus) | 🛒 (outline) | 🛒 (outline) |
| Tilapia (izumidai) | 🛒 (outline) | 🛒 (outline) |
| Toro (bluefin) | 🛒 (filled) | 🛒 (filled) |
| Unagi (freshwater eel) | 🛒 (filled) | 🛒 (filled) |
| Uni (sea urchin) | 🛒 (outline) | 🛒 (outline) |

My son Hunter and I gathered our lightest rods one morning when it was still dark and drove to Marina del Rey in Los Angeles to go sportfishing on the *Betty-O*, the same blue-and-white party boat my friends and I used to spend our weekends on from the time we were in junior high until I went away to college. He had a lightweight fluorescent green rod-and-reel combo prefilled with about a ten-pound test line, the kind of gear you buy at CVS, better suited for freshwater perch and crappie but making the fight with a big saltwater fish more of a contest. He knew already about DDT. It had leaked out from me over time as he learned what I do for what passes for a living. So, I figured, he kind of understood we would do catch-and-release.

"That's why we're using light tackle," I told him as we drove down the coast highway. "It's the fight that counts, you know?"

He looked at me at kind of a weird angle.

"What if it's a sea bass, Dad? You think we're not going to eat that? I don't think so."

I pulled onto Ocean Drive.

"Aren't there any fish we can eat from the bay?" he insisted.

"Okay, we catch a sea bass, we bring it home."

He side-eyed me.

It was a hit-and-miss day. Someone did hook into an early morning silvery sea bass that exploded from the thick inky soup and arched as it dove back into the sea. The man beside us fishing the bottom brought in a couple of barely legal spiny rockfish. They were maybe a half-inch past the legal limit. Hunter finally hooked solidly into a barracuda.

He followed his fish around the perimeter of the boat, patiently keeping tension but not too much, everyone yelling encouragement, the line going out, my son pumping, reeling in, adjusting his drag, filament taut, everyone expecting the line to snap until the streamlined white body surfaced.

Hunter brought the fanged, splashing fish close to the hull. My intent was to get a picture with my smartphone and cut the line to let it go. But one of the crew leaned down over the rail and gaffed its white underbelly, and now the fish flopped weakly, bleeding, turning the blue sea red.

Everyone around Hunter congratulated him on the fight and how he brought in the big one. I grabbed my smartphone and snapped Hunter in his broad-brimmed western hat with green rod-and-reel against his chest, cradling the long-jawed, toothy ten-pounder in his arms. He had this Clint Eastwood steely kind of glint in one picture and could have been the kid in a Normal Rockwell painting about to bring home his whopper for the family meal in another. Either way, I was so proud of my kid as he held the silvery barracuda in both arms across his chest.

"What should we do with him, Dad? I mean, if we're not going to eat him."

"Hey, you guys, if you don't want your fish, I'll take it," offered the red-faced, bearded man who had been bottom-fishing beside us.

His belly busted out of an extra-small T-shirt washed about one thousand times until it was so thin you could see through it.

"I'll take what you catch."

"Are you sure?" I said. "It might have some DDT."

"You think it's in these fish?"

"Yeah, I do."

He shook his head. "Man, it's everywhere, but I got five kids at home. I live in Hawaiian Gardens, you know where that is?" I nodded. "I didn't do nearly as well as I wanted today." He shook open his sack so I could look down at the bottom. "See, I got only two little bitty fishes."

My lips got tight.

"Can I give him the fish, Dad?" Hunter asked.

"Sure, go ahead," I barely got out.

I felt badly about what he was bringing home. I didn't like it, this feeling: his kids had to eat the contaminated catch from the bay and mine didn't. It seemed so unjust. But he really wanted the fish. He *needed* the fish.

"You fought this *hombre* beautifully," he told Hunter, taking the long, slender barracuda my son handed him.

The gulls gathered all around us, landing on the water and the ship's white-speckled railing. Sunlight dappled the sea. The man dropped the fish into his sack and walked away out of hearing distance.

"I hope his kids are going to be okay," Hunter said quietly.

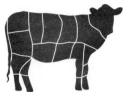

# Chapter 3

# Where's the Beef?

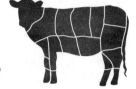

Mel Coleman Jr., in his thirties, wearing chaps over blue jeans, boots, brown cowboy hat, rawhide gloves, and bundled up against the cold winds, rode Buckskin, a sturdy, tanned, compact pony with a white blaze down the middle of his face. Mel Jr. had the same square, strong-jawed look of his father, who rode beside him. They rode their hoses at eight thousand feet elevation where the forests of spruce, pine, and aspen thinned, and eagles and hawks flew over the gray, slate-colored peaks, ringed with snow, worn down by brooks and streams that babbled down into the green meadows below. The cool moist breeze blew ripples through the wavering grass. The scene was from right out of the movies.

The two men breathed in deeply and gazed out upon a sprinkling of solid black cattle, spread out over the golden lands. The family ranched three thousand head of Angus beef. A lot of the ranches worked with Angus strains. But what made the Coleman family different than most of the other ranches was how they raised their cattle. They used pasture rotation with strategically placed water sources and fencing and took their cattle to higher elevations or into the range lands for their entire lives instead of overcrowding them in the bottoms of the valleys, causing environmental damage to pastures and waterways.

The Coleman ranch has long been headquartered in the northwest San Luis Valley, bordering the town of Saguache, Colorado, population 493, at an elevation of nearly 8,000 feet.

By the 1980s, the ranch included 17,000 deeded acres that had been part of the family since before 1876 or were acquired after that year, when Colorado received American statehood. The Coleman family leased nearly 3,000 acres from the US Forest Service and Department of Interior's Bureau of Land Management, located all the way back in Washington, D.C.

"The pasture rotation system we used actually increased grass density and improved wildlife habitat," Mel Jr. said proudly. "The fences were installed to provide pastures that could be grazed and then left alone. Over time, grass and wildlife increased and the watershed improved. Dad called the way we did things regenerative: as grassland managers, we worked with the rays of the sun and a little bit of rainfall to produce beef."

High inflation hit Americans in the late 1970s throughout the early 1980s. Money became too expensive to borrow. Beef was simply a commodity. The way the system worked, the ranchers were the last to profit. Some of the San Luis Valley family ranches, along with many in the West, were forced to liquidate their holdings. Still other families lost their ranches to the banks. The Colemans, like so many families, desperately sought a way to hold onto their ranch.

Help came from Mel Jr.'s brother and sister-in-law, who lived in Boulder and attended the University of Colorado.

"They told Dad some of their college friends as well as many of the Boulderites there wanted beef from cattle raised without antibiotics or added growth hormones," Mel Jr. remembered. "Dad asked them where they shopped, and they said at the natural food stores. Dad said, 'Good, we can do that. We'll call it "natural beef."' We marked our first production with a 'natural' stamp, which angered the US Department of Agriculture (USDA) local plant inspector. Dad hadn't realized *all* those labels and stamps that were on products needed USDA approval. The inspector in charge threatened to arrest him. Can you believe it? They said they'd throw him in jail for labeling his beef 'natural.' Imagine that! The most pure beef in the world, raised on grass, at an average elevation of nine thousand feet, and my dad couldn't call it 'natural.'

"Well, Dad went to Washington, D.C. many times after that and worked with USDA officials to develop a memorandum of understanding or MOU that would define the term 'natural.' That was the first time in the history of the nation beef was officially labeled natural."

Soon, demand outstripped supply. To meet the needs of their growing market, the family began working with a network of like-minded ranchers from Colorado and other Rocky Mountain states who were willing to raise their cattle under the Coleman Natural program standards.

"Dad became a voice for sustainability, which today is often referred to as 'regenerative agriculture and ranching,' sharing what he believed, experienced, and learned from working with ranchers and farmers throughout the country,"

Mel Jr. told me with a mixture of pride—and sadness over what became of the legal definition of what it meant to be "natural."

"Pressure from the chemical and drug companies and other industry players destroyed how 'natural' is defined," Mel Jr. went on. "They pressured USDA officials to revise the original 'natural' guidelines that covered how livestock is raised to just how meat is processed. Instead of covering how the animals were raised, fed, and treated, officials altered the regulations to make all fresh and processed meat 'natural' if it was minimally processed and contained no added artificial ingredients. However, the livestock industry was now free to use synthetic sex hormones, growth stimulants, and subtherapeutic antibiotics. I do think, overall, the USDA inspection service has done a great job in protecting consumers. Our disappointment with them was changing the original definition of 'natural,' limiting its meaning to how meat is processed.

"Dad—as I do—cared about how our livestock are raised and treated. By branding our meats, we let consumers know how our animals are raised, handled, and treated. Coleman program producers we're partnering with now in the rural Midwest are interested in sustainability and working hard to pass on their farms and ranches to the next generation. They want them to stay in the family. When people see the Coleman logo today on their beef and pork products, they know what it stands for. It means each animal was cared about and lived their lives naturally and humanely.

"I think now, more than ever, that's one of the things I've focused on. I want our customers to know Coleman products are coming from local, rural family farms. These are family farmers and ranchers who care just like you do."

I tested Coleman beef and found it was DDT-free. But, on the other hand, I also know that beef and other meats, when unwisely chosen, can become one of the major sources of DDT and other estrogenic organochlorine (OC) pesticides, synthetic hormones, and antibiotic residues in a child's diet. I know this might sound strange to some people. After all, DDT was banned in the 1970s. But the OCs are so persistent, durable, and fat soluble, they persist in soils in which grains are grown and accumulate in the fatty tissues of the cattle. These continue to be passed on, if present, from cow to calf.[1]

Making matters worse, factory-farmed cattle are also implanted with synthetic versions of the sex hormones: testosterone, estrogen, and progesterone.

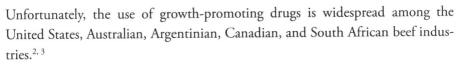
Unfortunately, the use of growth-promoting drugs is widespread among the United States, Australian, Argentinian, Canadian, and South African beef industries.[2, 3]

The combination of OCs and added sex hormones is why high-beef diets are associated with young girls reaching earlier menarche.[4] Early age at menarche opens the "estrogen window" for a longer time. This raises their breast cancer risk.[5]

Boys of mothers who eat high amounts of beef during pregnancy are at risk, too. They tend to have more cases of hypospadia (misplaced penile opening) and reduced sperm counts, both indicators of hormonal imbalances and feminization.[6, 7, 8]

## Where's the Beef?—A Family Protection Plan

Bison, chicken, turkey, and lamb are all raised without added growth-stimulating hormones. With the exception of lamb, they're usually leaner, have fewer OCs, and generally safer.

Pork, however, is likely to contain residues of sulfa drugs and growth stimulants. One commonly used drug, ractopamine, interferes with the endocrine system and stimulates tumor growth.[9, 10, 11, 12] Brands like Coleman Natural Foods have established longtime standards that avoid use of antibiotics, sulfa drugs, and growth stimulants when raising livestock.

American Grassfed Association (AGA) certification is the gold standard for all ruminant animals including bison, beef, sheep, dairy, goats, and hogs. The AGA is a nonprofit organization dedicated to supporting grassfed and pasture-based farmers. Its seal guarantees the farm animals lived their lives free and foraging until harvest without being given antibiotics and hormones.

Another indicator of safe flesh foods is USDA organic certification, which ensures farm animals are raised under humane conditions and their natural behaviors are accommodated; fed organic feed and forage; and free from antibiotics and synthetic hormones.

As I mentioned, my own tests of grassfed beef found no DDT. I also tested bison, which was DDT-free. Mammavation, a reliable online source for safe-shopping information, purchased and tested ButcherBox Organic Chicken and grassfed beef and found them to have nondetectable amounts of DDT too.[13]

I know, in this case, it's more expensive to buy grassfed or organic beef. But it's important during pregnancy and childhood to do so. You can also substitute safe, flesh- and plant-based protein sources such as chicken, turkey, or veggie burgers and hot dogs.

Plant-based meat substitutes, even if not organic, are better than the usual hormone-laden all-beef burger patty. But try to get organically sourced products when possible to avoid exposure to OP pesticides sprayed on the grains, legumes, and veggies used to make them.

I worry about processed meats cured with nitrite such as hot dogs, bologna, pepperoni pizza, and beef sticks, or that moms might consume them during pregnancy.

Once in the child's body, nitrite combines with chemicals called "amines" to form nitrosamines and raise their cancer risk. Cured meat consumption is particularly dangerous during pregnancy and strongly predicts a higher risk for childhood cancer.[14, 15]

You will see a lot of products whose labeling states they have no added nitrite and are uncured. These products include celery seed extract instead of nitrite. I definitely prefer these products when I do buy the kids cured and processed meats like sausages, hot dogs, and bologna, but with a caveat.

No one I've consulted is sure substituting celery seed extract actually makes cured meat any safer. Celery seed contains nitrate, which is inert. Nitrate must be converted to nitrite in order for it to become reactive and form carcinogenic nitrosamines. Some experts say celery seed's nitrate presents an equivalent risk to nitrite. Others argue the phytochemicals in the celery seed extract could inhibit the formation of nitrate into nitrite. The answer may be products with celery seed extract are safer. But by how much? This is an instance where we really do need more studies.

Go easy on processed meats with nitrite or celery seed extract; avoid during pregnancy; and, whenever possible, substitute safer choices instead of feeding them to your kids.[16]

# Safe and Unsafe Flesh Foods

| = Safe, none, or least risk from chemical toxins |
| = Dangerous, contains significant amounts of chemical toxins |
| All cuts are conventionally sourced unless otherwise noted |

| Food | Reproductive and Developmental Toxicity | Cancer |
|---|---|---|
| Beef (ground) | ⊘ | ⊘ |
| Beef ground, grassfed, organic | ✓ | ✓ |
| Beef loin/sirloin | ⊘ | ⊘ |
| Beef loin/sirloin, grassfed, organic | ✓ | ✓ |
| Beef chuck roast | ⊘ | ⊘ |
| Beef chuck roast, grassfed, organic | ✓ | ✓ |
| Bison | ✓ | ✓ |
| Bologna beef/pork, nitrite | ⊘ | ⊘ |
| Bologna beef/pork, nitrite-free, grassfed, organic* | ✓ | ✓ |
| Bologna chicken, nitrite | ⊘ | ⊘ |
| Bologna chicken, nitrite-free, grassfed, organic* | ✓ | ✓ |
| Bologna, tofu | ✓ | ✓ |
| Bologna, turkey, nitrite | ⊘ | ⊘ |
| Bologna, turkey, nitrite-free, grassfed, organic* | ✓ | ✓ |
| Chicken, drumsticks and breasts, breaded and fried, homemade | ⊘ | ⊘ |
| Chicken, drumsticks and breasts, breaded and fried, homemade, organic | ✓ | ✓ |
| Ham, cured, not canned, baked | ⊘ | ⊘ |
| Hot dog, beef, pork, nitrite | ⊘ | ⊘ |
| Hot dog, beef, pork, nitrite-free, grassfed, organic* | ✓ | ✓ |

*(Continued on next page)*

| Food | Reproductive and Developmental Toxicity | Cancer |
|---|---|---|
| Hot dog, chicken, turkey, nitrite | ● | ● |
| Hot dog, chicken, turkey, nitrite-free, grassfed, organic* | 🛒 | 🛒 |
| Hot dog, tofu | 🛒 | 🛒 |
| Lamb chop, pan-cooked with oil | ● | ● |
| Lamb chop, pan-cooked with oil, grassfed, organic | 🛒 | 🛒 |
| Liver beef/calf, pan-cooked with oil | ● | ● |
| Liver beef/calf, pan-cooked with oil, grassfed, organic | 🛒 | 🛒 |
| Meatloaf, beef, homemade | ● | ● |
| Meatloaf, beef, homemade, grassfed, organic | 🛒 | 🛒 |
| Pork bacon, oven-cooked, nitrite | ● | ● |
| Pork bacon, oven-cooked, nitrite-free, grassfed, organic* | 🛒 | 🛒 |
| Pork chop, pan-cooked with oil | ● | ● |
| Pork chop, pan-cooked with oil, grassfed, organic | 🛒 | 🛒 |
| Pork roast, loin, oven-roasted | ● | ● |
| Pork roast, loin, oven-roasted, grassfed, organic | 🛒 | 🛒 |
| Pork sausage link/patty, oven-cooked, nitrite | ● | ● |
| Pork sausage link/patty, oven-cooked, nitrite-free, grassfed, organic* | 🛒 | 🛒 |
| Salami, luncheon meat type not hard, nitrite | ● | ● |
| Salami, luncheon meat type not hard, nitrite, grassfed, organic* | 🛒 | 🛒 |
| Turkey breast, oven-roasted | 🛒 | 🛒 |
| Turkey breast, oven-roasted, organic | 🛒 | 🛒 |

* These foods may contain celery seed extract as a preservative, which hasn't been proven safe. Limit to once weekly.

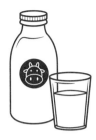

# Chapter 4

# Dairy on a Diet

Twelve hundred miles west of Saguache, Colorado, along the shores of the Pacific Ocean, above Tomales Bay, in Marin County, is the Straus Dairy Farm, whose cows have grazed on these lands since 1941.

Between 1940 and 1997, the number of dairy farms in the United States decreased 97 percent.[1] By 2017, the country had only 30,373 small commercial farms with fewer than two hundred cows. There had been 146,685 three decades before (in 1987).[2]

The same shrinkage occurred among the West Marin and Sonoma County dairy farmers of Northern California. Albert Straus, who had grown up on the family dairy farm, had the vision of inventive agricultural practices that were good for the planet, economically viable, and critical to the survival of small-scale farms. In 1994, Albert converted the family farm to organic. The same year, he founded Straus Family Creamery. With the emergence of the nation's first completely certified organic creamery, Albert created a market in the western United States that hadn't existed, finally giving consumers the opportunity to choose a healthy dairy product.

Albert explained to me: "Regenerative dairy farming is also known as carbon farming. It helps move carbon from the atmosphere and put it back into the soil. Herds are rotated to different pastures to improve productivity and stimulate plant growth while promoting soil health and regenerative practices. This intensive rotational grazing allows cows to eat high-quality grasses. Cows grazing on pasture minimizes weed intrusion and allows ample time for regrowth."

But at three cows per acre, the certified organic milk produced at the Straus Dairy Farm wasn't enough to meet their growing demand.

Today, Straus Family Creamery buys certified organic milk from twelve other local farms who care as much as you do about the food they produce.

Our nation continues to lose small dairy farms at an alarming rate, and most milk products come from factory farms where animals are routinely medicated with antibiotics to keep them healthy enough to continuously calve and lactate. Growth hormone is also injected into milk cows to increase production.

The more milk dairy herds are made to produce, the higher the incidence of conditions such as mastitis and other illnesses, requiring antibiotic medications that leave trace residues behind in the final product.

Antibiotic residues in milk and other dairy products have profound and wide-ranging impacts on a child's health. We've all heard about the human microbiome—all those beneficial and harmful bacterial colonies of life that reside in the gut. Children need to maintain a healthy biome in their gut in order to fight obesity, diabetes, cancer, and even for maintaining mental health. Yet, dairy products with antibiotics disrupt the intestine and kill a wide range of bacteria, including the good ones that keep the disease-causing organisms in check.[3] Conventionally sourced dairy also causes some bacteria to become antibiotic-resistant, rendering our usual medicines useless. Residues of antibiotics further weaken the child's cells by mutating the genes and damaging the structures of the DNA and RNA strands in their chromosomes. Chronic exposure to low-level antibiotics can also cause birth defects.[4]

About 10 to 20 percent of US dairy cows are injected with bovine growth hormone (BGH) to boost milk production.[5] Such milk need not be identified on labels. Yet, the amount of insulin-like growth-I factor can increase as much as sixfold in the milk from cows injected with BGH.[6] These higher exposures in women may play a role in stimulating breast cancer cells to metastasize.[7]

Regular whole dairy also has a lot of pesticide residues. As with fatty beef products, whole-milk dairy products contain traces of organochlorine (OC) pesticide residues, another alarming finding.

The OC pesticides build up in the fatty portions of dairy. As I've mentioned, the OCs are endocrine disruptors. They act like fake estrogens in the human body, feminize the male reproductive system, and cause hypospadia (misplaced penile opening), cancer, and autism.

Conventional whole-milk dairy products combine all three exposures—antibiotics, hormones, and the OC pesticides—in every glass.

# Dairy on a Diet—A Family Protection Plan

Rest easy. Do not let your mind be troubled by all of these chemical toxins. You can take smart steps to shield your children from the harmful contaminants in dairy products.

The big idea when shopping for dairy, whether conventionally or organically sourced, is to buy nonfat.

As with beef, OCs build up in the fatty portions. Nonfat milk, yogurt, sour cream, butter, cheese, cottage cheese, and other dairy are pesticide-free. This will be true whether the dairy is from organically raised or factory-farmed cows.

Also, even if you're not buying organic dairy, at least be sure somewhere on the carton that there's a "BGH-Free" statement. Kraft Foods, Starbucks, and Walmart have refused to sell milk products from BGH-treated cows.

Also, consider plant-based milks derived from oats, coconut, almonds, soy, and other sustainable, organically grown sources.

It's important to note factory-farmed eggs are likely to have residues of veterinary drugs that are needed when hens are kept in crowded, confined, and unnatural conditions. Most hens are still kept in cruel battery cages under dim lights in order to increase egg production.

"Battery cages are small, drawer-shaped cages a few feet wide and only about 15 inches tall—barely taller than the hens themselves," notes the Humane League.[8] "Depending on the size of the cage, between 4 and 10 birds are held in each cage. Industry guidelines recommend each bird having 67 to 86 square inches of space, which amounts to roughly the same space as a piece of lined paper."

Try to find eggs at least from cage-free farms, even if not organic. This is not by any means optimal, as hens may still be crowded and aren't afforded natural living conditions that allow for flight and other normal everyday activities. But cage-free is still a big improvement.

The most humane source for your family's eggs is "pasture-raised," which means chickens have access to the outdoors for many hours every day.

Animal Welfare Approved is run by A Greener World and guarantees hens can enjoy the great outdoors for their entire lives. The label also audits transport and slaughter practices and sends auditors to farms every year to ensure full ongoing compliance with standards.

Certified Humane cage-free eggs mean that hens were provided with 1.5 square feet of space per bird, as well as dust-bathing opportunities, perches, and better air quality. For free-range, hens must be given at least six hours of outdoor access every day, along with two square feet of space per hen when outdoors.

American Humane certifies cage-free, free-range, and pasture-raised eggs. Cage-free barns must provide scratching and dust-bathing opportunities. Free-range must have daytime access to outdoors that provides at least 21.8 square feet per hen. Pasture-raised hens must be given 108.9 square feet of outdoor access.

## Safe and Unsafe Dairy and Eggs

🛒 = Safe, none, or least risk from chemical toxins

🛒 = Dangerous, contains significant amounts of chemical toxins

All foods are sourced from conventionally raised animals unless otherwise noted

| Food | Reproductive and Developmental Toxicity | Cancer |
|---|---|---|
| Butter, regular (salted) | 🛒 | 🛒 |
| Butter, regular (salted), grassfed, organic | 🛒 | 🛒 |
| Cheese, American, processed | 🛒 | 🛒 |
| Cheese, American, processed, grassfed, organic | 🛒 | 🛒 |
| Cheese, cheddar, natural (sharp/mild) | 🛒 | 🛒 |
| Cheese, cheddar, natural (sharp/mild), organic | 🛒 | 🛒 |
| Cheese, Swiss, natural | 🛒 | 🛒 |
| Cheese, Swiss, natural, partly skim milk, | 🛒 | 🛒 |
| Cheese, Swiss, natural, partly skim milk, grassfed, organic | 🛒 | 🛒 |
| Cottage cheese, creamed 4% milk fat | 🛒 | 🛒 |
| Cottage cheese, creamed 4% milk fat, grassfed, organic | 🛒 | 🛒 |
| Cottage cheese, creamed, low-fat 2% milk fat | 🛒 | 🛒 |

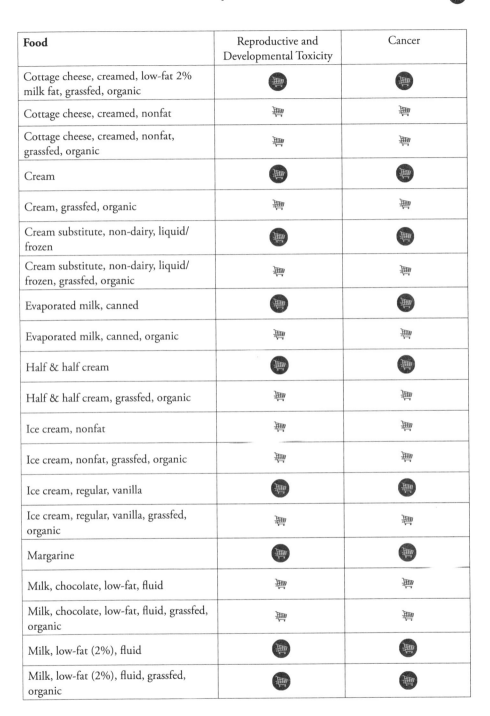

| Food | Reproductive and Developmental Toxicity | Cancer |
|---|---|---|
| Cottage cheese, creamed, low-fat 2% milk fat, grassfed, organic | 🛒 | 🛒 |
| Cottage cheese, creamed, nonfat | 🛒 | 🛒 |
| Cottage cheese, creamed, nonfat, grassfed, organic | 🛒 | 🛒 |
| Cream | 🛒 | 🛒 |
| Cream, grassfed, organic | 🛒 | 🛒 |
| Cream substitute, non-dairy, liquid/frozen | 🛒 | 🛒 |
| Cream substitute, non-dairy, liquid/frozen, grassfed, organic | 🛒 | 🛒 |
| Evaporated milk, canned | 🛒 | 🛒 |
| Evaporated milk, canned, organic | 🛒 | 🛒 |
| Half & half cream | 🛒 | 🛒 |
| Half & half cream, grassfed, organic | 🛒 | 🛒 |
| Ice cream, nonfat | 🛒 | 🛒 |
| Ice cream, nonfat, grassfed, organic | 🛒 | 🛒 |
| Ice cream, regular, vanilla | 🛒 | 🛒 |
| Ice cream, regular, vanilla, grassfed, organic | 🛒 | 🛒 |
| Margarine | 🛒 | 🛒 |
| Milk, chocolate, low-fat, fluid | 🛒 | 🛒 |
| Milk, chocolate, low-fat, fluid, grassfed, organic | 🛒 | 🛒 |
| Milk, low-fat (2%), fluid | 🛒 | 🛒 |
| Milk, low-fat (2%), fluid, grassfed, organic | 🛒 | 🛒 |

*(Continued on next page)*

| Food | Reproductive and Developmental Toxicity | Cancer |
|---|:---:|:---:|
| Milk, skim, fluid | 🛒 | 🛒 |
| Milk, skim, fluid, grassfed, organic | 🛒 | 🛒 |
| Milk, whole, fluid | 🛒 | 🛒 |
| Milk, whole, fluid, grassfed, organic | 🛒 | 🛒 |
| Sour cream, whole milk | 🛒 | 🛒 |
| Sour cream, grassfed, organic | 🛒 | 🛒 |
| Sour cream, nonfat | 🛒 | 🛒 |
| Sour cream dip, any flavor | 🛒 | 🛒 |
| Sour cream dip, any flavor, grassfed, organic | 🛒 | 🛒 |
| Yogurt plain, low-fat | 🛒 | 🛒 |
| Yogurt plain, low-fat, grassfed, organic | 🛒 | 🛒 |
| Yogurt, low-fat, fruit-flavored | 🛒 | 🛒 |
| Yogurt, low-fat, fruit-flavored, grassfed, organic | 🛒 | 🛒 |

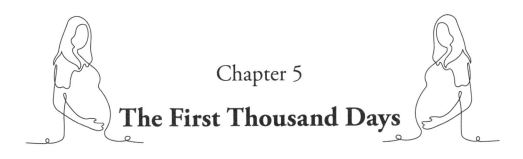

# Chapter 5
# The First Thousand Days

When Angela Sutherland became pregnant with her first child, she spent months researching nutrition. She discovered scientists considered the first thousand days—the period between the start of a woman's pregnancy and her child's second birthday—one of the most important and unique developmental periods.

Angela was also aware of reports that pesticides and heavy metals were being discovered in baby foods and dangerous to children's long-term health and neurological development. As a busy working mom, she lacked the time to make her own homemade baby food, but the jarred and overly processed products on store shelves had such long use-by dates that weren't appealing.

Fresh would be great. Fresh direct would be even better. But fresh direct wasn't anywhere to be found. Having graduated with a degree in mathematics from Brown University in Providence, Rhode Island, with a stint at Goldman Sachs, Angela was able to structure the private funding for an innovative new company that would do baby food differently.

In 2017, Angela, pregnant with her second child, together with her longtime friend, Evelyn Rusli, a writer for *The New York Times,* cofounded Yumi. The company delivers fresh, certified organic baby food to your doorstep throughout the country.[1]

"With Yumi, we wanted to make it easier to feed your baby fresh, delicious, nutrient-dense food," Angela said. "I'm proud of the way we're changing the conversation around childhood nutrition and impacting our customers' lives on a daily basis."

Yumi also endorsed the Baby Food Safety Act that Democratic senators introduced into Congress in 2022.[2] The proposed legislation wasn't passed. However, it would have set new lower limits for lead, mercury, arsenic, and cadmium contained in baby food and required manufacturers to regularly test and verify their products were meeting the new standards.

Because the proposed legislation never passed, however, parents shopping for baby foods need to be even more alert to potentially dangerous choices that might have high amounts of heavy metals and chemical toxins.

## The First Thousand Days— A Family Protection Plan

Keep in mind these big ideas when shopping for conventionally sourced baby foods:

- Rice is a leading source of pesticide-related arsenic exposure in the diet.[3] Use a frozen banana for teething, instead of a rice-based biscuit, to lower exposure. Yumi products are free of rice, and the company offers a rice-free organic Meltable Puff.
- Beef with gravy, broth, vegetables, macaroni, or tomatoes is laced with DDT. Dishes with turkey and chicken will always be safer than any with beef, according to the Food and Drug Administration (FDA) Total Diet Study. Serenity Kids has come out with ethically sourced bison and turkey formulas. Their products are more expensive, but bison and turkey are so much less toxic choices when your infant consumes flesh foods.
- Jarred sweet potato contains dicloran, which has been shown to cause testicular and uterine cancers.[4, 5, 6] Creamed spinach is high in DDT, according to the Total Diet Study.
- Applesauce and juice, peaches, pears, and mixed fruit are filled with organophosphate nerve toxins. Definitely go for organic fruits.

Onceuponafarm.com is a source of organic fruit juices and blends. The baby-food company is the brainchild of actor Jennifer Garner, whose own century-old family farm, located in Locust Grove, Oklahoma, produces some of the organic fruits and veggies for their plant-based meals and cold-pressed blends.

The Healthy Living Foundation (HLF) found high amounts of an industrial chemical called acrylamide, a carcinogen and reproductive toxin, in Earth's Best Gluten-Free Broccoli Cheese Nuggets. The HLF has taken legal action against

Earth's Best parent company Hain Celestial Group. The amounts were very high, according to independent testing. In our legal action, we allege this product is unsafe for toddlers and infants and violates the California health and safety code. I'll take a deep dive into this industrial chemical's presence in kids' snack foods in chapter 8.

But, for now, you should be aware of these brands: Nabisco Arrowroot and Gerber Butter biscuits, Parent's Choice Baked Apple Grahams, and Plum Organics Little Yums Teething Pumpkin & Banana Wafers were the heaviest acrylamide carriers, according to FDA testing.

On the other hand, organically sourced Happy Baby, Happy Tot, and O Organics dishes were acrylamide-free.

## Safe and Unsafe Baby Foods

🛒 = Safe, none, or least risk from chemical toxins

🛒(dark) = Dangerous, contains significant amounts of chemical toxins

All foods are conventionally grown unless otherwise noted

| Food | Reproductive and Developmental Toxicity | Cancer |
| --- | --- | --- |
| Apple juice | Dangerous | Dangerous |
| Applesauce | Dangerous | Dangerous |
| Beef and broth/gravy | Dangerous | Dangerous |
| Beef and vegetables | Dangerous | Dangerous |
| Carrots | Safe | Safe |
| Chicken and broth/gravy | Safe | Safe |
| Chicken and vegetables | Safe | Safe |
| Chicken noodle dinner | Safe | Safe |
| Creamed corn | Safe | Safe |
| Creamed spinach | Dangerous | Dangerous |
| Fruit dessert/pudding | Dangerous | Dangerous |

*(Continued on next page)*

| Food | Reproductive and Developmental Toxicity | Cancer |
|---|:---:|:---:|
| Green beans | 🛒 | 🛒 |
| Ham and vegetables | 🛒 | 🛒 |
| Infant formula, milk-based, high RTF | 🛒 | 🛒 |
| Infant formula, milk-based, low iron, ready to feed | 🛒 | 🛒 |
| Macaroni, tomato, and beef | 🛒 | 🛒 |
| Mixed vegetables | 🛒 | 🛒 |
| Orange juice | 🛒 | 🛒 |
| Peaches | 🛒 | 🛒 |
| Peas | 🛒 | 🛒 |
| Sweet potatoes | 🛒 | 🛒 |
| Turkey and rice | 🛒 | 🛒 |
| Vanilla custard/pudding | 🛒 | 🛒 |
| Vegetables and beef | 🛒 | 🛒 |
| Vegetables and chicken | 🛒 | 🛒 |
| Vegetables and ham | 🛒 | 🛒 |

# Safe and Unsafe Baby Food Brands Tested for Acrylamide

| Product | Amount of Acrylamide (in parts per billion) ND = Non-detectable | Toxicity Rating |
|---|---|---|
| Beech-Nut Rice Cereal for Baby | ND | 🛒 |
| Beech-Nut Stage 1 Oatmeal Cereal for Baby | ND | 🛒 |
| Beech-Nut Stage 2 Apples & Cherries | ND | 🛒 |
| Beech-Nut Stage 2 Butternut Squash | 22 | 🛒 |
| Beech-Nut Stage 2 Carrots & Peas | 17 | 🛒 |
| Beech-Nut Stage 2 Tender Golden Sweet Potatoes | 37 | 🛒 |
| Beech-Nut Stage 2 Vegetables & Chicken | 75 | 🛒 |
| Beech-Nut Classics Stage 2 Corn & Sweet Potato | ND | 🛒 |
| Beech-Nut Stage 2 Banana, Orange & Pineapple | ND | 🛒 |
| Carnation Baby Cereal with Formula Oatmeal | ND | 🛒 |
| Carnation Baby Cereal with Formula Rice | ND | 🛒 |
| Comforts for Toddler Strawberry Yogurt Puffs | 730 | 🛒 |
| Earth's Best Chicken Nuggets | ND | 🛒 |
| Earth's Best Gluten Free Nuggets with Broccoli and Cheese | 568 | 🛒 |
| Earth's Best Organic Apple Peach Oatmeal Fruit & Grain Puree | ND | 🛒 |
| Earth's Best Organic Stage 2 Apples & Apricots | ND | 🛒 |
| Earth's Best Organic Stage 2 Carrots | ND | 🛒 |
| Earth's Best Organic Sweet Potato Apple Baby Food Puree | ND | 🛒 |
| Ella's Kitchen Apples + Strawberries | ND | 🛒 |
| Ella's Kitchen Pears Peas + Broccoli | ND | 🛒 |
| Ella's Kitchen Toddler Oat + Honey Cookies | 50 | 🛒 |
| Full Circle Organic Stage 2 Mixed Vegetables | 40 | 🛒 |

*(Continued on next page)*

59

| Product | Amount of Acrylamide (in parts per billion) ND = Non-detectable | Toxicity Rating |
|---|---|---|
| Gerber 1st Foods Sweet Potatoes | ND | 🛒 |
| Gerber 2nd Foods Apples & Cherries | ND | 🛒 |
| Gerber 2nd Foods Carrots & Sweet Potatoes | 39 | 🛒 |
| Gerber 2nd Foods Chicken Dinner | 30 | 🛒 |
| Gerber 2nd Foods Green Beans | 26 | 🛒 |
| Gerber 2nd Foods Pears | ND | 🛒 |
| Gerber 2nd Foods Squash | ND | 🛒 |
| Gerber 2nd Foods Sweet Potatoes | 68 | 🛒 |
| Gerber Finger Food Butter Biscuits | 130 | 🛒 |
| Gerber Finger Food Fruit Wagon Wheels | 20 | 🛒 |
| Gerber Graduates for Toddlers Animal Crackers | 60 | 🛒 |
| Gerber Graduates Lil' Biscuits Vanilla Wheat | ND | 🛒 |
| Gerber Graduates Puffs Peach | 50 | 🛒 |
| Gerber Mixed Cereal for Baby | ND | 🛒 |
| Gerber Single Grain Oatmeal Cereal for Baby | ND | 🛒 |
| Gerber Tender Harvest Organic Sweet Potatoes | 92 | 🛒 |
| Happy Baby Gentle Teethers Banana and Sweet Potato | ND | 🛒 |
| Happy Baby Gentle Teethers Blueberry & Purple Carrot Teething Wafers | ND | 🛒 |
| Happy Baby Organic Puffs Purple Carrot & Blueberry | ND | 🛒 |
| Happy Tot Best Friends Toddler Cookies Chocolate Pumpkin | 60 | 🛒 |
| Happy Tot Sweet Potato, Apple, Carrot & Cinnamon | ND | 🛒 |
| Hot-Kid Baby Mum-Mum Apple Rice Rusks | 410 | 🛒 |

| Product | Amount of Acrylamide (in parts per billion) ND = Non-detectable | Toxicity Rating |
|---|---|---|
| Meijer Baby Apple Rice Rusks | 27 | 🛒 |
| Meijer Baby Little Puffs Banana | 30 | 🛒 |
| Nabisco Arrowroot Biscuit | 113 | 🛒 |
| Nabisco Zwieback Toast | 20 | 🛒 |
| O Organics Stage 2 Applesauce | ND | 🛒 |
| O Organics Stage 2 Summer Vegetables | ND | 🛒 |
| Parent's Choice Toddler Baked Graham Cookies Apple | 420 | 🛒 |
| Parent's Choice Toddler Squeezable Fruit Banana, Apple & Blueberry | ND | 🛒 |
| Plum Organics Just Mangos Organic Stage 1 Baby Food | ND | 🛒 |
| Plum Organics Little Yums Organic Teething Wafers Pumpkin & Banana | 220 | 🛒 |
| Plum Organics Super Puffs Blueberry & Purple Sweet Potato | ND | 🛒 |
| Sprout Organic Baby Food Stage 2 Sweet Potato, White Beans & Cinnamon | 20 | 🛒 |
| Tippy Toes Stage 2 Apple Banana | ND | 🛒 |
| Tippy Toes Stage 2 Apple Pear Banana | ND | 🛒 |
| Wild Harvest Organic Stage 2 Sweet Potatoes | 10 | 🛒 |

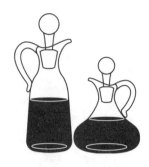

# Chapter 6

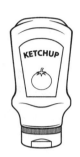

# The Extras

How did so much of the organochlorine (OC) pesticides, lindane, benzene hexachloride (BHC), and endosulfan—all endocrine disruptors, the first two long banned—get into the yellow mustard spread on my kids' hot dog buns? And why are there residues of another banned OC, dieldrin, in their pickles?

Dad (a.k.a. nerd avenger) went to work. The answer was that lindane (along with its environmental breakdown byproduct BHC) was sprayed on the Brassicaceae seeds (from which mustard is made) before being banned in countries such as China, a major global exporter, only in 2019.[1, 2] Its residues continue to contaminate agricultural soils. Dieldrin, on the other hand, has proven so durable that, although banned in many nations for some half a century, it continues to persist, for some reason, in agricultural soils where cucumbers are grown, which is why traces of it show up in dill and sour pickles.[3] Plants' roots absorb these residues systemically. Processing concentrates them.

Tomato ketchup is a steady source of OCs, too. But in this case, endosulfan, yet another OC pesticide, is still being applied to tomatoes (as well as those mustard seedlings).

Conventionally grown black olives are sprayed with dicofol, an OC fungicide with DDT, as part of its standard mixture.

Be wary of your olive oil as well. It might be time for a change if you buy California Olive Ranch, America's most popular (although industrially produced) brand of this ancient elixir. Testing done by independent laboratories for the Healthy Living Foundation (HLF) found the product was contaminated with the highly potent sperm toxin carbaryl, which is banned for almost all uses in California, New York, Canada, and the European Union, and harms male reproductive health. The HLF filed a lawsuit against California Olive Ranch and several major supermarket chains when they failed to inform consumers about the presence of this harmful, banned chemical toxin in their olive-oil products.

Most worrying: epidemiological studies performed by Dr. John Meeker, senior associate dean for research, University of Michigan School of Public Health, show sperm damage occurs in infertile men at normal dietary exposures.[4] Low-level exposures are also thought to cause poor female egg quality.[5]

Exposure to carbaryl during pregnancy is associated with developmental disabilities in young children.[6] Knowingly dosing pregnant people daily with carbaryl-contaminated olive oil—or persons of childbearing age who want to start a family but are finding it difficult—without informing them first, constitutes a toxic assault against California's citizens. The company's actions, in the HLF's view, clearly violate the Safe Drinking Water and Toxic Enforcement Act, the public health law requiring just such information be provided to the consumer prior to purchase.

California Olive Ranch, despite being repeatedly and urgently informed by our group through filing multiple notices of violation with the State Attorney General and served to the company, as well, has refused up to this day to inform consumers who buy their product about the presence of carbaryl and, in my mind, clearly put profits over people's health.

In California, the people have a right to know about this powerful reproductive toxin's repeated presence in such an important daily dietary staple.

## The Extras—A Family Protection Plan

They may be the extras. But they add up.

Make condiments organic whenever possible.

But if you do buy conventionally sourced condiments and dressings, ensure they are nonfat whenever possible to avoid exposure to the OC pesticides. Be aware: low-calorie isn't the same as low-fat. Look for dressings stating they're nonfat.

Make sure your olive oil is organically sourced (unlike California Olive Ranch). Simple Truth is an economic organic olive oil. In contrast to California Olive Ranch, the HLF's independent testing found Bertolli's and Vesuvius olive oils free from more than one hundred different pesticide residues including carbaryl.

# Safe and Unsafe Condiments, Dressings, and Oils

 = Safe, none, or least risk from chemical toxins

 = Dangerous, contains significant amounts of chemical toxins

All foods are conventionally grown unless otherwise noted

| Food | Reproductive and Developmental Toxicity | Cancer |
|---|:---:|:---:|
| Bertolli's Olive Oil |  |  |
| Black olives |  |  |
| Black olives, organic |  |  |
| Brown gravy, canned or bottled |  |  |
| Brown gravy, homemade |  |  |
| California Olive Ranch oil |  |  |
| Cream substitute, non-dairy, liquid/ frozen |  |  |
| French salad dressing, regular |  |  |
| Honey |  |  |
| Honey, organic |  |  |
| Italian salad dressing, low-calorie |  |  |
| Mayonnaise, regular, bottled |  |  |
| Mayonnaise, regular, bottled, organic |  |  |
| Olive oil, non-organic |  |  |
| Olive oil, organic |  |  |
| Pancake syrup |  |  |
| Relish |  |  |
| Relish, organic |  |  |

| Food | Reproductive and Developmental Toxicity | Cancer |
|---|---|---|
| Salad dressing, creamy/buttermilk type, low-calorie | 🛒 | 🛒 |
| Salad dressing, creamy/buttermilk type, regular | 🛒 | 🛒 |
| Sweet cucumber pickles | ⬤🛒 | ⬤🛒 |
| Sweet cucumber pickles, organic | 🛒 | 🛒 |
| Tomato ketchup | ⬤🛒 | ⬤🛒 |
| Tomato ketchup, organic | 🛒 | 🛒 |
| Vegetable oil | 🛒 | 🛒 |
| Vesuvius Olive Oil | 🛒 | 🛒 |
| Yellow mustard | ⬤🛒 | ⬤🛒 |
| Yellow mustard, organic | 🛒 | 🛒 |

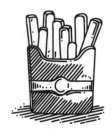
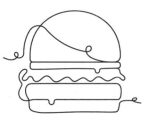

# Chapter 7

# Dark Side of a Happy Meal

So how was it that I came to be lost, somewhere off of California Highway 101 in the Salinas Valley, with three starving kids, seeking someplace safe to eat late at night that wouldn't make me feel like I'd completely violated everything in which I believed?

"I should have brought along enough sandwiches," I told my partner upon leaving the whitewashed adobe walls of the Spanish Mission San Antonio de Padua, situated in the middle of miles and miles of sandy valley land.

Learning about our state's history was part of the twins' fourth-grade curriculum—but there were certainly no restaurants, stores, gas stations, or rest stops. Just that mission in my rearview mirror . . . and a carload of hungry cubs.

It was dusty; wind gusts rocked Rupert, our black 1999 4-Runner with grills over its lights, back and forth, carrying us back toward civilization.

"We're so hungry, Dad," Sharla, my eight-year-old daughter, moaned.

"Let's get Indian food," said Spense, my oldest.

"Yeah, curry in a hurry," chimed Hunter.

"Do we have any water?" Sharla called.

"I should have brought along more water too," I added wistfully.

"That's called kid-trip mismanagement," my partner laughed.

We lumbered into Soledad. The spotlights of the local state prison glowed eastward and illuminated the distant mountain slopes like the backdrop of a black-and-white film.

The brightly glowering, glimmering signage of McDonald's, Burger King, Taco Bell, and Wendy's lured us into the fast-food jungle.

I was certain I was the only parent in the world making fast-food decisions for their kids based on chemical toxicity as much as nutrition. I drove slowly, keeping a keen eye out for a safe harbor.

Despite my sense of isolation, 7 in 10 parents are concerned about the presence of unsafe chemicals in what their children eat, according to a report in *Food Safety News*.[1]

No wonder it's a parental topic of hot concern. We're worrying more, but our kids are eating less healthily. What's going on? More than one-third of children and teens eat fast food on any given day.[2] The total daily percentage of calories from fast food our kids take in increased from almost 11 percent in 2009 to more than 14 percent by 2018.

Kids consume more hormones, per- and polyfluoroalkyl substances (PFAS), toluene, benzene, phthalates, and bisphenols than ever before thanks to fast food.[3, 4]

One thing is for sure, fast-food beef is some of the worst in the world. Almost all of the beef for chains such as McDonald's and Wendy's is "from cattle ranches right here in North America," which, considering that cattle in the United States are routinely raised with added hormones, I don't find reassuring in any sense.[5, 6] The same goes for take-out beef tacos, tostadas, and fast-food sandwiches.

Eating fast food numbs children to the horrors of factory farming and distorts their sense of right and wrong. We know in our heart of hearts that farm animals deserve to be treated humanely. But fast food is the ultimate stealth desensitizer, so much inhumanity to animals slipping past the child's brain right to the gut. I see a fast-food kids' meal as the ultimate concentration of all of the horrors of industrialized agriculture and factory farming, compressed into a single beef patty of indeterminate estrogenicity (due to synthetic hormones) fit between two slices of a distinctly unnatural white bun, loaded with organophosphate (OP) pesticide nerve toxins that were developed from chemical warfare weapons in Germany in the 1930s.

With some 386 chemical residues detected in 44 samples in the Food and Drug Administration (FDA) Total Diet Study, the all-American favorite, a quarter pounder with cheese, barely beats out a plain quarter pounder for the most toxic fast food.

Each bite of a quarter pounder with cheese had some 8.7 chemical residues, including relatively high amounts of pesticides such as DDT and its related compounds, which act like the female hormone estrogen in the human body. Just getting a plain quarter pounder won't help much either, as these samples had only 14 fewer toxic residues.

With 334 chemical traces found in 44 samples, including pesticides and traces of packaging materials, beef tacos and tostadas were nearly as contaminated as a quarter pounder, according to the same FDA study.

"Dad, did you hear me? We're starving!" Sharla cried out.

"Is there an In-N-Out around here?" Hunter said.

We found a green and yellow sign that screamed Subway. It wasn't perfect but wasn't, to my mind, the disaster McDonald's or Taco Bell would be if we went there.

We trooped inside, huddled up against the cold wind.

Hunter wanted the cold-cut combo, but the meat was cured with nitrite. As I noted in chapter 3, nitrite is converted into cancerous nitrosamines. Sharla chose the B.M.T. (which stands for bigger, meatier, tastier, I learned). Nitrite was present there, too. Spenser wanted to go with turkey, a smart choice. I did tuna. My partner went vegetarian. But at that time, that meant pretty much a salad on bread.

The kids yielded to my swift attempt at an educational sermon and ended up getting tuna, turkey, and chicken breast, all nitrite-free. The veggies were better than fries any day or night. The bread was one foot of enriched flour, which (I suspected) contained OP pesticides. I did get the kids to order Swiss cheese partially made with nonfat milk. Also, no fatty dressing. They got their sandwiches with sliced avocado, oil, and vinegar, all relatively safer.

Once back on Highway 101, leaving behind the valley, we rose in elevation. The mountains were all around us. The cubs were asleep. My partner was smiling, and everything was okay.

All I had to do was drive well and get them safely home that last stretch of winding highway.

## Dark Side of a Happy Meal— A Family Protection Plan

We know all of the worst stops along the fast-food highway. These guidelines below will shine a light on all of the safe ones.

Do you have a Shake Shack yet in your community? **Shake Shack** has 377 fast-casual-dining restaurants throughout North America and globally.[7] They're publicly committed to humane farming and sourcing flesh foods from animals raised without hormones and antibiotics.

**Burgerfi** is also adamant about humane farming practices that include no added hormones. They have 120 locations including drive-throughs, many in the South.[8]

**Chick-fil-A** may be known for its original hand-breaded chicken sandwich; thankfully, they offer grilled menu items that come with salad (instead of fries).

My kids are **El Pollo Loco** fans. They like their barbecued rotisserie chicken more than beef, anyway. The beans beat fries hands down any day for a low-toxin side. The beans and tortillas are not organic (not yet, at least) but with salsa they could well offer a healthy low-toxin lunch or dinner fiesta.

**Panera Bread** and **Chipotle**, both with thousands of locations, are additional low-toxin choices. Both companies say their humane-farming guidelines exclude use of antibiotics, hormones, and other growth stimulants. Chipotle sources organically grown ingredients "when possible."[9]

Maybe just try to get the kids to order Chinese fast food. Chow mein with beef or chicken, beef with vegetables, and chicken with vegetables are by far safer than any of the typical fast foods, according to the Total Diet Study.

But what if you're halfway between Salinas and Paso Robles (like I was) with a desperately starving backseat crew?

If you've got to pull in *someplace*, here are some easy ways to make sure your kids eat as healthily and safely as possible for the rest of your drive home.

***Substitute with poultry.*** No hormones are approved for use in raising poultry in the United States. Poultry is also leaner, which means fewer fat-loving chemicals like DDT. Turkey is even more pure than chicken, according to the FDA Total Diet Study.

***Go plant-based.*** Burger King's Impossible Burger appears so real (they say, not me), "the patties appear to bleed like a real cow," according to *Business Insider*.[10]

Carl's Jr.'s charbroiled Beyond Burger patty is an alternative to the usual toxic jungle beef. They're not organic, but their DDT load is much lower, and they don't have synthetic hormones.

***Ditch the nuggets.*** It's difficult to pull into a McDonald's or Burger King and get grilled flesh foods like chicken or fish. But, whenever possible, choose grilled over battered. All that batter is an OP pesticide sop. Chicken nuggets were contaminated with 266 toxic chemical residues in 44 Total Diet Study samples. A quarter of them were OP pesticides sprayed on the grains used for the flour in the batter for the crust. A fish sandwich (battered), with 199 residues in 44 samples, isn't pretty. But don't blame the poor haddock. A great proportion of those residues are from the chemical toxins in the flour. No fast-food chicken or fish should be consumed battered.

***Give French fries to the enemy.*** French fries round out the top most toxic fast foods with 321 chemicals in 44 samples, or some 7 in each "cancer stick," a slang reference to cigarettes. In addition to pesticides, fast-food fries are a source of the industrial carcinogen acrylamide. You will learn why acrylamide is particularly harmful to our daughters in chapter 8. But, for now, if all that fat and those empty calories aren't enough to make you deny your kids, consider the number of pesticides and that an industrial chemical also contaminates them. No caring parent could give their kids one of these.

French fries from Popeyes and Fuddruckers are the worst when it comes to acrylamide levels, according to FDA tests. If the kids are craving fries, try to divert their attention. Tell them "French fries" is actually an American term. The French themselves do not refer to the dish as such and are truly a lean nation. Do whatever it takes to make it home where you can bake them one of the safer homemade products that I'll share with you in chapter 8.

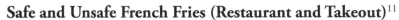

# Safe and Unsafe French Fries (Restaurant and Takeout)[11]

| Product | Amount of Acrylamide (in parts per billion) ND = Non-detectable | Toxic Rating |
|---|---|---|
| Applebee's French Fries | 940 | 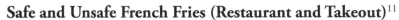 |
| Applebee's Sweet Potato Fries | 880 | 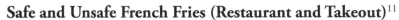 |
| Arby's | 252 | 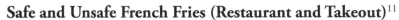 |
| Big Al's Gourmet Butter-Made Burgers Sweet Potato Fries | 940 | 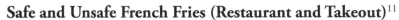 |
| Braum's Crinkle Cut French Fries | 250 | 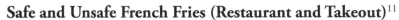 |
| Burger King | 262 | 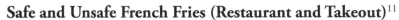 |
| Checkers | 332 | 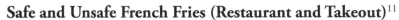 |
| Chick-fil-A | 389 | 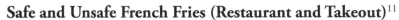 |
| Colton's Steak House Baked Potato | 200 | 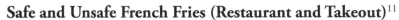 |
| Colton's Steak House Baked Sweet Potato | 90 | 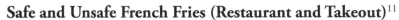 |
| Colton's Steak House Sweet Potato Fries | 640 | 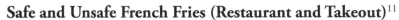 |
| Colton's Steak House Trail Potatoes Potato Skins | 1440 | 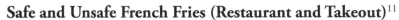 |
| Cracker Barrel Hash Browns | 460 | 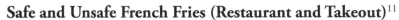 |
| Dixie Cafe Baked Potato | 110 | 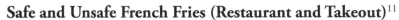 |
| Dixie Cafe French Fries | 290 | 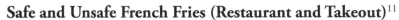 |
| Fuddruckers Wedge Cut-Fries | 399 | 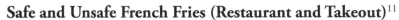 |
| Golden Corral Baked Potato | 10 | 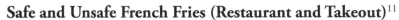 |
| Grub Burger Bar Sweet Potato Fries | 1020 | 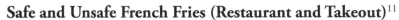 |
| Huddle House French Fries | 280 | 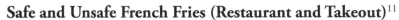 |
| IHOP French Fries | 560 | 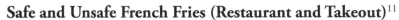 |
| IHOP Hash Browns | 1090 | 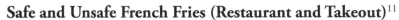 |

*(Continued on next page)*

| Product | Amount of Acrylamide (in parts per billion) ND = Non-detectable | Toxic Rating |
|---|---|---|
| J&J's Scoreboard Bar & Grill Potato Skins | 780 | 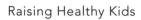 |
| J&J's Scoreboard Bar & Grill Sweet Potato Tots | 700 | |
| KFC Fries | 216 | |
| Logan's Roadhouse Loaded Potato Skins | 1330 | |
| Logan's Roadhouse Baked Potato | ND | |
| Logan's Roadhouse Baked Sweet Potato | 250 | |
| LongHorn Steakhouse Sweet Potato | 70 | |
| McDonald's Fries | 388 | |
| Outback Steakhouse Aussie Fries | 940 | |
| Outback Steakhouse Sweet Potato with Honey Butter & Brown Sugar | 60 | |
| Perkins Restaurant & Bakery Baked Potato | 150 | |
| Perkins Restaurant & Bakery Hash Browns | 410 | |
| Popeyes Fries | 606 | |
| Red Robin Sweet Potato Fries | 1030 | |
| Smashburger Sweet Potato Fries | 860 | |
| Smokin' Joes Sweet Potato Fries | 930 | |
| Sonic Natural-Cut Fries | 300 | |
| Texas Land & Cattle Steakhouse Baked Sweet Potato | 370 | |
| Tuttle's French Fries | 370 | |
| Tuttle's Sweet Potato Fries | 320 | |
| Village Inn Hash Browns | 560 | |
| Waffle House Hash Browns | 1260 | |

| Product | Amount of Acrylamide (in parts per billion) ND = Non-detectable | Toxic Rating |
|---|---|---|
| Wendy's French Fries | 228 | |
| Woody's Grille Seasoned Waffle Fries | 610 | |
| Woody's Grille Sweet Potato Fries | 940 | |

Brenda Hampton grew up in the town of Courtland, Alabama, along the Tennessee River, downstream from Decatur, in Lawrence County. There was once a time her stretch of the river was home to more than one hundred varieties of freshwater mussels. A diver could make five hundred dollars a day harvesting them.

But, in the 1960s, 3M set up a massive plant along the river that began manufacturing products using PFAS.[12] Among these was fast-food packaging. The PFAS made materials resistant to grease and moisture. Trouble was, they were also killers, and they began assaulting the life in the waters of the river and then the people.

"The mussels all but disappeared by the 1990s," Brenda told me. "Many of the divers who once made a living from harvesting them have long passed or are still dying in their sixties and seventies from river cancer."

Brenda's children, nieces, and nephews—and many persons throughout the whole town—began experiencing kidney disease and cancer.

"It seemed like there was a new kidney dialysis clinic popping up on every corner," Brenda told me.

It wasn't until 2016 Brenda learned her home's water had been contaminated with PFAS for over forty years. The upstream plant, which was using PFAS for manufacturing oil-, heat-, and moisture-resistant fast-food containers, was contaminating the river that provided her family with their drinking water.

In 2018, she joined with the nonprofit activist groups Toxic-Free Future and Change.org, shared her story online, and the public responded with seventy-five thousand signatures for a petition demanding McDonald's stop using PFAS in their packaging. McDonald's finally relented in 2022 and promised to stop using these dangerous chemicals by 2025. That's two slow-moving years away as I write.

How much PFAS is in our kids' bodies from fast-food containers? That depends on how many fast-food and restaurant meals they enjoy—and which establishments you patronize.

One study found levels of PFAS in human blood were much higher after feasting on fast food and take-out pizza than from persons who ate their meals at home.[13]

*Consumer Reports* surveyed fast-food packaging in 2021 in Connecticut, Mississippi, New Jersey, New York, and Texas for total organic fluorine, a marker for PFAS chemicals, and published their results in 2022.[14] In 2023, the state of California banned food packaging with PFAS that exceed 100 parts per million (ppm). However, *Consumer Reports* notes that food packaging with amounts of PFAS at 20 ppm or less meets "a stricter standard . . . set by Denmark." *Consumer Reports* "supports that lower cutoff." For more information on this *Consumer Reports* survey, please see the appendix on page 205.

## *Can Carry-Out and Delivery Be Healthier?*

Bring your own containers (BYOC) when you do takeout. Use stainless-steel or polypropylene takeout containers instead of the styrene and PFAS-infused ones you still usually get.

California legislation gives consumers the right to bring reusable takeout containers into restaurants and temporary food-service facilities at events. Most restaurants value your business and are happy to accept your containers. A restaurant or carry-out kit can consist of stainless-steel food containers, mugs, and reusable utensils. MIRA makes stainless-steel carriers. I also have reusable mugs in our car for the kids when we order hot and cold takeout beverages.

Deliverzero.com is the go-to website for the growing **network of conscientious takeout and restaurant delivery services offering** reusable, PFAS-free containers. (They're generally used one thousand or more times instead of single-use toxic takeout containers.)[15]

Foreverware.org partners with eateries in Minnesota, Illinois, Wisconsin, Ohio, and New Hampshire to supply takeout in reusable, PFAS-free containers.

I've rated the top fast-food brands in the nation, from best to worst, to help make it easier for you the next time you're in the middle of almost nowhere, the kids are famished, and you've got to get them *something*.

# Safe and Unsafe Fast-Food Brands (from best to worst)

| Company | Comments |
| --- | --- |
| **Shake Shack** | Hormone-free beef with humane farming methods; committed to no PFAS. |
| **Sweetgreen** | No PFAS, organic greens. Locally sourced. Nearly 1000 locations in the US including California, Texas, New York, and Florida plus the UK.[16] |
| **Chipotle** | Committed to organic and no-hormone, humanely raised beef and flesh foods. Committed to no PFAS.[17] |
| **Chick-fil-A** | Grilled chicken with salads make much lower toxin choices.[18] Customers can order the chain's first organic menu option, Honest Kids® Appley Ever After® juice drink, as part of the Chick-fil-A Kid's Meal in restaurants nationwide.[19] |
| **El Pollo Loco** | Uses some organic ingredients, Mexican dishes that reduce chemical toxins. |
| **Panera** | Serves antibiotic- and cage-free poultry. Some 89% or more of beef is from grassfed cattle. Pork is sourced from gestation crate-free farms. Committed to PFAS-free packaging. Limited commitment to organically sourced ingredients.[20] |
| **BurgerFi** | No hormones, humanely raised beef. The restaurants and drive-throughs are committed to no PFAS. |
| **Subway** | Some nitrite- and preservative-free cold cuts. No PFAS. The chain's animal welfare standards are too broad and vague.[21] The bread and veggies aren't organic (which is bad) but better than their competitors' fries when it's late at night. |
| **White Castle** | Offers the Impossible Slider, a plant-based alternative to their famous sliders, with a dairy-free alternative to cheddar cheese. No published standards for PFAS, humane animal treatment, or use of synthetic hormones. |
| **Jack in the Box** | PFAS-free packaging as of 2023.[22] Some 77 percent of its eggs come from cage-free chickens.[23] No policy restricting antibiotic- or hormone-use in beef and poultry.[24] |
| **Wendy's** | Uses antibiotic- and hormone-treated flesh foods.[25] Committed to elimination of PFAS only from consumer-facing packaging. Testing confirms low or none.[26] |
| **Five Guys** | Uses hormone-treated beef. Hot dogs are cured with nitrite.[27] |
| **Burger King** | Uses hormone-treated beef. Committed to phasing out PFAS by 2025.[28] |
| **Tim Hortons** | Uses Canadian beef, which is given synthetic hormones. Committed to phasing out PFAS by 2025 but has received failing grades for packaging safety in the meantime.[29] |

*(Continued on next page)*

| Company | Comments |
|---------|----------|
| Popeyes | Committed to phasing out PFAS by 2025.[30] However, the chain uses conventionally sourced flour for its batter and crust. |
| Carl's Junior | Uses hormone-treated beef. |
| In-N-Out | Uses hormone-treated beef.[31] |
| McDonald's | Uses hormone-treated beef. Has committed to gradual removal of PFAS from packaging. |

My daughter, Sharla, brought home Shake Shack burgers for us to share the other day. A lot of what we tell our kids when they're teens seems to make no impression on them. Then, one day, they surprise you.

She put them on the table, and our muddy-pawed collie dogs gathered around, taking their usual spots, placing their black-and-white snouts into strategic positions, looking up at us with sympathetic eyes. That burger, dripping with juice, piled with sweet onions, was wonderful.

And yes, the boys got theirs too. In fact, they're always first (and last).

"You got Shake Shack?" I said to Sharla with a mixture of surprise and pride.

"Yeah, after you telling us that we were going to get all contaminated by the burgers we really love, I thought I'd get these. I figured it would make you happy and cut short the lecture."

"And if you were getting a burger for yourself?" I said.

Sharla took a bite of the burger.

"Well, I'd definitely give this another try."

Sometimes, fathers and mothers really do know best. And trust the collies. They know a good burger when they taste one!

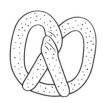 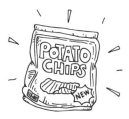

# Chapter 8

# Worse than Cigarette Smoke

Our twins, Hunter and Sharla, were sixteen when they did the shopping for their first Super Bowl Sunday to watch the Patriots face the Eagles in February 2018. All evening, I heard the sounds of them and their friends flipping tops off of soft drinks, ripping open bags of chips, cheering, and jeering as the game went back and forth. That was the year the Eagles handed Patriots quarterback Tom Brady one of his rare Super Bowl losses.

Sharla and I ended cleaning up after everyone left, sweeping the floor, wiping salsa off the walls (not sure how it got there), dabbing the formerly unstained white couch with a nontoxic, enzyme-based spot remover, gathering wrappers, jars, boxes, and bowls bearing the colorful lettering of Chex, Pepperidge Farm, Trader Joe's, and Justin's.

"I'm glad y'all are so into healthy foods," I laughed, holding a bag of Chex Spicy Jalapeno Cheddar Snack Mix.

"We got healthy food, too, Dad," Sharla countered.

She twisted the lid back on the top of a bottle of Justin's Classic Almond Nut Butter and held it up proudly.

"Nut butter is totally Paleo," she said. "Wasn't that a good shopping choice?"

"I don't know," I replied in a low, plaintive drawl.

"What do you mean? I heard Justin's is supposed to be really environmentally conscious."

"Yeah, I know what they *say*, darling. But I'm studying snack foods. I want to test nut butters and those Chex snacks, too, for a toxic chemical called acrylamide."

"Why, Dad?"

"It causes cancer."

"Oh no," she said. "I feel bad now. I served it to everybody. I had some too, Dad. Is it going to hurt me?"

"Well, first, we don't know if there's even any in Justin's," I said. "Maybe it will have very low levels or none. So let's wait to find out, okay?"

"Shouldn't they tell us, like on the label or something?"

"Yes," I said. "I think so. A lot of people would like to know."

Sharla put the Justin's container in the palm of my hand as if she were a disobedient puppy.

"You didn't do anything wrong," I said.

I hugged her and brushed my hand through her hair.

"It's not your fault, sweetie. Don't worry," I told her.

"Just let me know when you get the verdict," she said.

I did.

She was shocked.

Swedish scientists' 2002 discovery of acrylamide in baked and snack foods helped solve another health mystery: why women in the industrialized world have experienced steep rises in endometrial (also known as uterine) and ovarian cancer. Acrylamide is an industrial chemical used in pigments and dyes. An all-around carcinogen and reproductive toxin, it's baked into foods when processors use poor-quality raw materials, combine the wrong ingredients, or rely on outdated processing methods involving needlessly high temperatures.

As if causing cancer wasn't bad enough, acrylamide is an endocrine disruptor. It fits like a key into the locks of the cell receptors on the surfaces of our daughters' estrogen-sensitive reproductive tissues. A natural estrogen molecule flips the gene switches on and off, does its job, and breaks down. But when synthetic acrylamide connects to the cell receptors, it works like a super virus or a mad gamer who can't keep their hands off the console.[1]

These powerful genetic mishaps cause our daughters to produce and metabolize exorbitant amounts of a form of high-octane, toxic estrogen that lasts longer in the body and stimulates endless rounds of cell division of the reproductive tissues. The cells of the uterus become deranged. They lose their ability to die naturally in a welcomed biological process called apoptosis. They just keep dividing. This overgrowth can begin to spread and form tumors.[2, 3, 4]

In one study among women in 2007, the risk for endometrial, ovarian, and breast cancer in the highest acrylamide-consuming group increased by

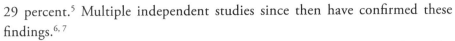

29 percent.[5] Multiple independent studies since then have confirmed these findings.[6, 7]

Fortunately, testing by the Food and Drug Administration (FDA) and Healthy Living Foundation (HLF) shows most companies have taken acrylamide's presence in snack foods seriously. The FDA has worked with the snack industry to voluntarily implement updated processing controls, and most companies have done an exemplary job of reducing the amount of acrylamide in their products. But in the course of the HLF's work as a toxic enforcer, our testing has also revealed some of the worst scofflaws.

This is important information, too. We parents have a manageable way to prevent endometrial cancer in our daughters. Eliminating acrylamide from the diet will reduce this known risk—especially by avoiding the worst offenders. It's that simple.

Reading labels is important but won't help with acrylamide. The presence of artificial sweeteners, food dyes, polysorbate, high-fructose corn syrup, and other added sugars on the label are a clear indicator such products shouldn't be on anybody's healthy shopping list or in their pantry. These additives are associated with childhood obesity, diabetes, anxiety disorder, ADHD, and cancer.[8]

Acrylamide, on the other hand, an established carcinogen and reproductive toxin, like cadmium and lead, isn't listed on any label, and it's not as if manufacturers and distributors with the worst products are going to voluntarily share with shoppers that their products contain the poison.

The Environmental Protection Agency regulates the amount of acrylamide in drinking water. But the FDA won't do the same for acrylamide in food products. Instead, it offers voluntary guidelines to manufacturers about how to reduce or eliminate the chemical's presence. But there are no federal standards and no requirements for disclosing when products have harmful amounts.

I found out how bad it can get when I received the lab results for Chex snack mixes and the amount of the acrylamide was so high the toxicologist who performed the cancer-risk assessment told us a child could consume them safely no more than three or four times a year. So much for packing Chex in kids' school lunches.

Justin's Classic Nut Butter harbored such a high, unsafe amount of the poison it could be eaten only three times a year before exceeding California's safe intake for acrylamide. It was by far the worst of all the nut butters the HLF tested. Thumbs-down to Justin's and Justin Gold, the company founder. No one who cares about kids would knowingly sell or promote this kind of dangerous product to our daughters.

I instructed our lawyers to sue Justin's, Chex, and Pepsico (for their HealthWise Protein Chips, also contaminated with high amounts of the industrial chemical), which they did once they saw the test results. The HLF also has taken legal action against Trader Joe's and Earth's Best for selling acrylamide- contaminated food products without label warnings intended for children. Watch out for these and other specific products detailed throughout this chapter.

In fact, I've curated results from HLF and FDA testing for the safe shopping charts in the rest of this chapter. This is the only way to get this information to you in a manner that's both educational and shopper-friendly.

## Worse than Cigarette Smoke— A Family Protection Plan

Keeping up with a family's insatiable snacking demands *and* eliminating major sources of acrylamide from their lives takes savvy substituting.

You've got to stay alert and take proactive actions to keep the cupboard, fridge, and freezer supplied with healthy, low-, or acrylamide-free snacks.

One thing's for sure: kids are more likely to snack on healthy fruits, veggies, and nuts if they're within arm's reach.

Here's what I suggest:

Keep a bowl of healthy nuts and dried fruit within arm's reach on the kitchen counter. Kids are impulsive. They'll reach for the bowl if it's what they see first. I keep one bowl filled with almonds, peanuts, cashews, walnuts, Brazil nuts, pumpkin and sunflower seeds, goji berries, raisins, cacao nibs, sliced dates, mangoes, pineapple, and other healthy tidbits that can be added to the mix so that it's always fresh and tasty. Make sure your nuts are unroasted, unsalted, and preferably organic.

I also place bowls of cut colorful veggies, nonfat or organic dips, and apples, oranges, and grapes in the front of the fridge at eye level so the kids will see them first.

Keep a never-ending supply of salsa, guacamole and healthy, low-acrylamide blue corn chips available at all hours.

Remove all poisonous products from your pantry.

Quinn, Rold Gold, and Shultz are safer choices than Chex.[9, 10, 11]

## Safe and Unsafe Pretzels

| Product | Amount of Acrylamide (in parts per billion) ND = Non-detectable | Toxic Rating (Levels below 70 ppb present least risk) |
|---|---|---|
| Always Save Mini Twist Pretzels | 140 | |
| Beigel & Beigel Pretzels Sesame Rings | 120 | |
| Chex Savory Bold Party Blend | **462** | |
| Chex Indulgent Dark Chocolate Snack Mix | **257** | |
| Chex Savory Cheddar Snack Mix | **441** | |
| Chex Traditional Snack Mix | **563** | |
| Chex Bold Party Blend | **909** | |
| First Street Mini Twist Pretzels | 233 | |
| Good Health Salted Peanut Butter Filled Pretzels | 138 | |
| Great Value Pretzel Sticks | 90 | |
| King Henry's Peanut Butter Pretzel Nuggets | 160 | |
| Kroger Pretzel Haus Stick Pretzels | 130 | |
| Nice! Mini Twist Pretzels | 110 | |
| Publix Thin Stick Pretzels | 90 | |
| Quinn | 20 | |
| Rold Gold Pretzel Sticks | 20 | |
| Shultz Stick Pretzels | 70 | |
| Snyder's of Hanover Sticks Pretzels | 90 | |

Pita bread and crackers, pizza crust, naan, and lavash are all generally safe choices. The faster-cooked flatbread, matzo—prepared as the Jews fled their Egyptian chains of slavery—is cherished for Passover and Saturday mornings.

Because it's truly baked more quickly at higher temperatures, matzo tends to have elevated acrylamide concentrations.[12] Since matzo is such an integral part of the Passover Seder meal, it's important to serve it, and eating it one holiday a year won't be unsafe. Just make this the exception. (After all, the Seder service asks, "Why is this night different from all other nights?") Refrain from snacking on matzo the rest of the year.

On the other hand, Essential Everyday, Giant Food, Haggen, Meijer, Nabisco, and Pepperidge Farm crackers have tested safe for year-round snacking.

## Safe and Unsafe Flatbread and Crackers

| Product | Amount of Acrylamide (in parts per billion) ND = Non-detectable | Toxic Rating (Levels below 70 ppb present least risk) |
| --- | --- | --- |
| Back to Nature Multigrain Flax Seeded Flatbread Crackers | 410 | |
| Cheez It Baked White Cheddar Snack Crackers | ND | |
| Essential Everyday Thin Wheat Crackers | ND | |
| Giant Food Baked Wheat Snack Crackers | ND | |
| Great Value Saltine Crackers | 100 | |
| Haggen Saltine Crackers Unsalted Tops | 50 | |
| Haggen Wheat Wafers Made From Whole Grain | 20 | |
| Homekist Saltines | 40 | |
| Mary's Gone Crackers Herb Crackers | 200 | |
| Meijer Apricot & Raisin Cracker Crisps | 60 | |
| Meijer Reduced Fat Baked Wheat Crackers | ND | |
| Nabisco Ritz Crackers | ND | |
| Nabisco Whole Grain Original Wheat Thins | 20 | |
| Pepperidge Farm Golden Butter Crackers | ND | |
| Pepperidge Farm Goldfish Baked Snack Cracker Pizza | ND | |

*(Continued on next page)*

| Product | Amount of Acrylamide (in parts per billion) ND = Non-detectable | Toxic Rating (Levels below 70 ppb present least risk) |
|---|---|---|
| Red Oval Farm Stoned Wheat Thins Wheat Crackers | 330 | |
| Rold Gold Thin Crisps Honey Dijon | 243 | |
| Safeway Kitchens Original Thin Wheat Baked Snack Crackers | 100 | |
| Safeway Kitchens Saltine Crackers | 60 | |
| Special Value Saltines | 60 | |
| Streit's Matzos Lightly Salted | 800 | |
| Sunshine Krispy Saltine Crackers | 50 | |
| Town House Flatbread Sea Salt & Olive Oil | 40 | |
| Trader Joe's Reduced Guilt Wheat Crisps | 50 | |
| Traders Joe's Fig & Olive Crisps | 350 | |
| Wasa Hearty Whole Grain Crispbread | 90 | |
| Weis Original Saltines | 40 | |

General Mills Corn Chex cereal delivers kids a knockout punch of acrylamide just like their snack packs. Wheatena cereal is an acrylamide sponge, according to FDA testing. Toss them.

The FDA's testing further shows that the lowest level cereals for acrylamide and pesticide exposures include Familia Original Recipes Swiss Muesli, Kashi Organic Promise Cinnamon Harvest, Malto-Meal, and Nature's Path Organic Whole O's. By the way, cereals made by boiling water on the stovetop or in the microwave oven are acrylamide-free.[13] Enjoy your instant oats!

# Safe and Unsafe Cereals

| Product | Amount of Acrylamide (in parts per billion) ND = Non-detectable | Toxic Rating (Levels below 70 ppb present least risk) |
|---|---|---|
| 365 Everyday Value Little Cubbies | ND | 🛒 |
| Anjou Bakery Provisions Company Crostini Fruit & Nut | 10 | 🛒 |
| Anjou Bakery Provisions Company Crostini Fruit & Nut | 20 | 🛒 |
| Back to Nature Multigrain Flax Seeded Flatbread Crackers | 400 | ⬤ |
| Best Choice Corn Flakes Cereal | 380 | ⬤ |
| Breadshop's Sierra Crunch Muesli | 51 | 🛒 |
| Clover Valley Corn Flakes | 360 | ⬤ |
| Essential Everyday Muesli with Raisins, Dates & Almonds | ND | 🛒 |
| Familia Original Recipes Swiss Muesli | 11 | 🛒 |
| Full Circle Organic Toasted Oats | ND | 🛒 |
| General Mills Cheerios | 266 | ⬤ |
| General Mills Cinnamon Toast Crunch | 61 | 🛒 |
| General Mills Corn Chex | 1210 | ⬤ |
| General Mills Honey Nut Cheerios | 146 | ⬤ |
| General Mills Lucky Charms | 176 | ⬤ |
| Great Value Corn Flakes | 110 | ⬤ |
| Health Valley Low-Fat Granola Tropical Fruit | 89 | ⬤ |
| Heartland Granola Cereal Original | 20 | 🛒 |
| Kashi Organic Promise Cinnamon Harvest | ND | 🛒 |
| Kellogg's Corn Flakes | 90 | ⬤ |
| Kellogg's Corn Pops | 71 | ⬤ |

*(Continued on next page)*

| Product | Amount of Acrylamide (in parts per billion) ND = Non-detectable | Toxic Rating (Levels below 70 ppb present least risk) |
|---|---|---|
| Kellogg's Frosted Flakes | 52 | 🛒 |
| Kellogg's Frosted Mini-Wheats | 78 | ⬤ |
| Kellogg's Mueslix Cereal with Raisins, Dates & Almonds | 28 | 🛒 |
| Kellogg's Raisin Bran | 156 | ⬤ |
| Kellogg's Rice Krispies | 47 | 🛒 |
| Kroger Frosted Toasted Oats with Marshmallows | 40 | 🛒 |
| Laura Lynn Shredded Wheat Bite Size | 40 | 🛒 |
| Malt O Meal Raisin Bran | 30 | 🛒 |
| Mom's Best Cereals Toasted Wheat-Fuls | 150 | ⬤ |
| Nature's Path Organic Whole O's | 10 | 🛒 |
| One Degree Veganic Sprouted Ancient Grain O's | 80 | 🛒 |
| Post Grape-Nuts | 67 | 🛒 |
| Post Honey Bunches of Oats Crunchy Honey Roasted | ND | 🛒 |
| Post Selects Great Grains, Raisins, Dates & Almonds | 30 | 🛒 |
| Quaker 100% Natural Granola Oats, Honey & Raisins | 84 | ⬤ |
| Quaker Simply Granola Oats, Honey, Raisins & Almonds | ND | 🛒 |
| Sunbelt Fruit & Nut Granola Cereal, Raisins, Dates & Almonds | 20 | 🛒 |
| The Silver Palate Grain Berry Bran Flakes | 70 | 🛒 |
| Trader Joe's Maple Pecan Clusters | 130 | ⬤ |
| Weightwatchers Oat Clusters with Almonds | ND | 🛒 |
| Wheatena Toasted Wheat Cereal | 1057 | ⬤ |
| Whole Foods Market 365 Oat Bran Flakes Cereal | 189 | ⬤ |

Pancakes are a safer choice than cereals and waffles. Van's, a popular nonorganic waffle brand, has high amounts of acrylamide. Market Pantry is the best nonorganic choice for waffles. I recommend organic pancakes and waffles, which are the same price as those made from conventionally sourced grains.

## Safe and Unsafe Pancakes and Waffles

| Product | Amount of Acrylamide (in parts per billion) ND = Non-detectable | Toxic Rating (Levels below 70 ppb present least risk) |
|---|---|---|
| Aunt Jemima Buttermilk Pancakes | 113 | 🛒 |
| Aunt Jemima Confetti Pancakes | 16 | 🛒 |
| Aunt Jemima French Toast | 16 | 🛒 |
| Aunt Jemima Homestyle Pancakes | 10 | 🛒 |
| Aunt Jemima Low Fat Pancakes | 13 | 🛒 |
| Bob Evans Breakfast Bakes Sausage, Egg, Cheese, & Hash Browns | 30 | 🛒 |
| Cracker Barrel Pancakes | 10 | 🛒 |
| De Wafelbakkers Buttermilk Pancakes | 27 | 🛒 |
| De Wafelbakkers Maple Pancakes | ND | 🛒 |
| Giant Brand Buttermilk Pancakes | ND | 🛒 |
| Giant Brand Extra Fluffy Waffles Belgian Style | ND | 🛒 |
| Giant Brand Pancakes Original | ND | 🛒 |
| Great Value Blueberry Waffles | 48 | 🛒 |
| Great Value Buttermilk Waffles | 68 | 🛒 |
| Great Value Homestyle Waffles | 87 | 🛒 |
| IHOP Buttermilk Pancakes | 10 | 🛒 |
| Kellogg's Eggo French Toaster Sticks Original | ND | 🛒 |
| Kellogg's Eggo Blueberry Waffles | 45 | 🛒 |
| Kellogg's Eggo Buttermilk Waffles | 37 | 🛒 |

*(Continued on next page)*

| Product | Amount of Acrylamide (in parts per billion) ND = Non-detectable | Toxic Rating (Levels below 70 ppb present least risk) |
|---|---|---|
| Kellogg's Eggo Chocolate Chip Waffles | 32 | 🛒 |
| Kellogg's Eggo French Toaster Sticks Original | 13 | 🛒 |
| Kellogg's Eggo Homestyle Waffles | 71 | 🛒 |
| Kellogg's Eggo Strawberry Waffles | 90 | 🛒 |
| Lucy's Diner Pancakes | ND | 🛒 |
| Market Pantry Blueberry Waffles | 29 | 🛒 |
| Market Pantry Buttermilk Waffles | 12 | 🛒 |
| Market Pantry Original French Toast | ND | 🛒 |
| Pillsbury Buttermilk Pancakes | 57 | 🛒 |
| Pillsbury Homestyle Pancakes | 84 | 🛒 |
| Van's 8 Whole Grains Multigrain Waffles | 174 | 🛒 |
| Van's Multigrain Belgian Waffles | 146 | 🛒 |
| Van's Gluten Free Apple Cinnamon Waffles | 258 | 🛒 |
| Van's Gluten Free Blueberry Waffles | 353 | 🛒 |
| Van's Gluten Free Cinnamon French Toast Sticks | 32 | 🛒 |
| Van's Gluten Free Waffles | 230 | 🛒 |
| Village Inn Multigrain Pancakes | 10 | 🛒 |
| Woody's Grille Buttermilk Pancakes | ND | 🛒 |

Potato chips' toxicity is off the charts.

But if you find you or your kids jonesing for them, Utz Home Style Kettle-Cooked has you covered.

# Safe and Unsafe Potato Chips

| Product | Amount of Acrylamide (in parts per billion) ND = Non-detectable | Toxic Rating (Levels below 70 ppb present least risk) |
|---|---|---|
| Always Save Original Potato Chips | 720 | 🛒 |
| Baked Lay's Potato Crisps | 693 | 🛒 |
| Better Made Potato Chips Original | 1370 | 🛒 |
| Cape Cod Kettle Cooked Potato Chips Original | 220 | 🛒 |
| Clover Valley Ripple Cut Potato Chips | 460 | 🛒 |
| Good Health Natural Foods Olive Oil Potato Chips Plain | 385 | 🛒 |
| Grandma Utz's Handcooked Potato Chips | 146 | 🛒 |
| Great Value Original Potato Chips | 760 | 🛒 |
| Guy's Original Potato Chips | 780 | 🛒 |
| Health Wise Protein Chips Barbecue Crunch | 450 | 🛒 |
| Health Wise Protein Chips Pizza Crunch | 580 | 🛒 |
| Health Wise Protein Chips Ranch Crunch | 530 | 🛒 |
| Herr's Crisp 'NB Tasty Potato Chips | 468 | 🛒 |
| Kettle Brand Real Sliced Potatoes Sea Salt | 430 | 🛒 |
| Kettle Chips Lightly Salted Natural Gourmet Potato Chips | 1265 | 🛒 |
| Kiddylicious Sweet Potato Crisps | ND | 🛒 |
| Lay's Classic Potato Chips | 1410 | 🛒 |
| Lay's Kettle Cooked Mesquite BBQ Flavored Potato Chips | 198 | 🛒 |
| Lay's Stax Potato Crisps Original | 530 | 🛒 |
| Lay's WOW! Original Potato Crisps | 415 | 🛒 |

*(Continued on next page)*

| Product | Amount of Acrylamide (in parts per billion) ND = Non-detectable | Toxic Rating (Levels below 70 ppb present least risk) |
|---|---|---|
| Lunds & Byerlys Kettle Chips Traditional | 290 | |
| Magic Original Potato Chips | 330 | |
| Michael Season's Thin & Crispy Lightly Salted Potato Chips | 1230 | |
| MiCostenita Papitas Casera Homemade Potatoes | 1770 | |
| Munchos Potato Crisps | 580 | |
| Old Dutch Potato Chips Original | 360 | |
| Pringles Original Potato Crisps | 570 | |
| Pringles Ridges Original Potato Chips | 1286 | |
| Pringles Sweet Mesquite BBQ Flavored Potato Crisps | 2510 | |
| Ruffles Original Potato Chips | 292 | |
| Ruffles Potato Chips Original | 170 | |
| Ruffles WOW! Original Potato Crisps | 270 | |
| Sensible Portions Garden Veggie Straws Zesty Ranch | 1270 | |
| Sweet Potato Chips with Sea Salt Crinkle Cut | 8440 | |
| Terra Sweet Potato Chips No Salt | 260 | |
| Tom's Original Potato Chips | 420 | |
| Utz Crisp All-Natural Potato chips | 656 | |
| Utz Home Style Kettle-Cooked Potato Chips | 117 | |
| Wavy Lay's Original Potato Chips | 198 | |
| Wise All Natural Potato Chips | 600 | |

Tortilla chips, anyone? Can you convince the kids to prefer tortilla chips served with salsa and guacamole? Blue corn chips with their higher antioxidants have the least amount of acrylamide.[14]

On the Border, Fritos, Tostitos Multigrain and Roasted Garlic & Black Bean, and Kroger are your safest choices.

Other alternatives made with beans, plantains, and other veggies have emerged in the marketplace, but some are so toxic they're flashing red. Plantain chips tested high in acrylamide. Eden, Kashi, Nabisco, and Primizie offer safer, lower-toxin alternatives.

Even that longtime American schoolyard trading premium, Frito Corn Chips, is a safer choice than potato chips.

## Safe and Unsafe Tortilla Chips, Etc.

| Product | Amount of Acrylamide (in parts per billion) ND = Non-detectable | Toxic Rating (Levels below 70 ppb present least risk) |
|---|---|---|
| Always Save Big Dipper Corn Chips | 410 | |
| Ara Real Plantain Chips | 740 | |
| Beanitos Original Black Bean Chips with Sea Salt | 103 | |
| Boulder Canyon Rice & Bean Snack Chips with Adzuki Beans | 70 | |
| Calbee Saya Snow Pea Crisps Original | 30 | |
| Calbee Shrimp Chips Baked | 107 | |
| Calidad Corn Tortilla Chips | 400 | |
| Chifles Plantain Chips | 320 | |
| Churrumais Fried Corn Strips Spicy Lemon | 280 | |
| Del Ranchito Original Pork Rinds | ND | |
| Eat Smart Snacks Veggie Crisps Sea Salt | 200 | |
| Eden Sea Vegetable Chips | ND | |

*(Continued on next page)*

| Product | Amount of Acrylamide (in parts per billion) ND = Non-detectable | Toxic Rating (Levels below 70 ppb present least risk) |
|---|---|---|
| Food Should Taste Good Multigrain Tortilla Chips | 120 | |
| Fritos Corn Chips | 30 | |
| Good & Delish Restaurant Style Multi-Grain Tortilla Chips | 160 | |
| Good Health Veggie Chips Sea Salt | 1050 | |
| Goya Plantain Chips | 360 | |
| Grace Green Banana Chips | 390 | |
| Great Value Corn Chips | 350 | |
| Kashi Caramelized Onion Hummus Crisps | 57 | |
| Kroger Corn Chips Original | 390 | |
| Kroger Private Selection Multigrain Tortilla Chips | 120 | |
| Late July Sea Salt Multigrain Tortilla Chips | 500 | |
| Levant Snack Foods Falafel Chips Original | 500 | |
| Mayté Plantains Strips | 150 | |
| Medallion Corn Chips Original Flavor | 350 | |
| Mediterranean Snacks Baked Lentil Chips Parmesan Garlic | 100 | |
| MiCostenita Wheat Pellets | ND | |
| Nabisco Wheat Thins Toasted Pita Original | 10 | |
| Nongshim Shrimp Crackers | 20 | |
| Nonni's Thin Addictives Pistachio Almond Thins | 50 | |
| Old London Bagel Chips Sea Salt | 200 | |
| On the Border Cantina Thins Tortilla Chips | 60 | |
| Party-Tizers Fiesta Bean Dippin' Chips Black, Red & Adzuki Beans | ND | |

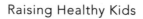

| Product | Amount of Acrylamide (in parts per billion) ND = Non-detectable | Toxic Rating (Levels below 70 ppb present least risk) |
|---|---|---|
| Popchips Potato Sea Salt | 3060 | |
| Primizie Thick Cut Crispbreads Classic Italian 7-Herb Blend | ND | |
| Publix Restaurant Style Tortilla Chips | 150 | |
| Samai Plantain Chips Pacific Sea Salt | 180 | |
| Sensible Portions Garden Veggie Chips | 510 | |
| Sensible Portions Garden Veggie Chips Sea Salt | 590 | |
| Sensible Portions Garden Veggie Chips Sour Cream & Onion | 160 | |
| Simple Truth Vegetable Chips | 300 | |
| Simply 7 Hummus Chips Sea Salt | 70 | |
| Simply Balanced Organic Rolled Tortilla Chips 7 Seeds & Grains | 610 | |
| Simply Sprouted Way Better Snacks Black Bean Corn Tortilla Chips | 180 | |
| Simply Sprouted Way Better Snacks Multi-Grain Corn Tortilla Chips | 160 | |
| Simply Sprouted Way Better Snacks Sweet Potato Corn Tortilla Chips | 610 | |
| Slim Jim Original Smoked Snack Stick | ND | |
| Snyder's of Hanover Reduced Fat Restaurant Style Tortilla Chips | 440 | |
| Soldanza Bananitos Lightly Salted Banana Chips | 120 | |
| Stacy's Pita Chips Simply Naked Sea Salt | ND | |
| Stark Smoki Flips | 80 | |
| Stobi Flips with Peanuts | 90 | |
| Sun Chips French Onion | 70 | |
| Terra Vegetable Chips Sea Salt | 370 | |

*(Continued on next page)*

| Product | Amount of Acrylamide (in parts per billion) ND = Non-detectable | Toxic Rating (Levels below 70 ppb present least risk) |
|---|---|---|
| The Real Deal Snacks Veggie Chips Original | ND | |
| Tostitos Cantina Traditional Tortilla Chips | 250 | |
| Tostitos Multigrain Scoops | 20 | |
| Tostitos Multigrain Tortilla Chips | 410 | |
| Tostitos Roasted Garlic & Black Bean Tortilla Chips | 30 | |
| Trader Joe's Quinoa and Black Bean Infused Tortilla Chips | 50 | |
| Xochitl White Corn Chips | 340 | |
| Terra Sweet Potato Chips No Salt | 260 | |

I know, I was pretty harsh when it came to fast-food French fries in chapter 7. Still, if you've gotten your kids to say no to them with the promise you will make them fries when you get home, there's good news: Alexia, McCain, Ore-Ida, and Wegmans offer safer choices.

## Safe and Unsafe Supermarket French Fries, Tater Rounds, and Hash Browns

| Product | Amount of Acrylamide (in parts per billion) ND = Non-detectable | Toxic Rating (Levels below 70 ppb present least risk) |
|---|---|---|
| 365 Everyday Value Crinkle Cut Sweet Potato Fries (baked) | 40 | |
| Alexia 98% Fat Free Smart Classics Roasted Crinkle Cut Fries (baked) | 150 | |
| Alexia Rib Cut BBQ Sweet Potato Fries With Skin On (baked) | 20 | |
| Alexia Rib Cut BBQ Sweet Potato Fries With Skin On (fried) | 20 | |
| Alexia Sweet Potato Fries | 160 | |
| Alexia Sweet Potato Fries Sea Salt | 60 | |

| Product | Amount of Acrylamide (in parts per billion) ND = Non-detectable | Toxic Rating (Levels below 70 ppb present least risk) |
|---|---|---|
| Alexia Sweet Potato Puffs (fried) | 120 | 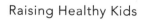 |
| Earthbound Farm Roasted Organic Sweet Potato Slices Sea Salt & Olive Oil | 130 | |
| Giant Brand Extra Crispy Crinkle Cut French Fried Potatoes | 100 | |
| Giant Brand Extra Crispy Fried Potatoes | 70 | |
| Giant Brand O'Brien Style Hash Browns | 1290 | |
| Giant Brand Seasoned Fries | 110 | |
| Giant Brand Tater Bites | 400 | |
| Lamb Weston Inland Valley French Fries | 212 | |
| Linden Farms French Fries Shoestring Style | 70 | |
| McCain Baby Cakes Hash Browns | 353 | |
| McCain Craft Beer Batter Fries | ND | |
| McCain Craft Beer Battered Potatoes Thin Cut Fries | 30 | |
| McCain Crinkle Cut | 49 | |
| McCain Home Style Baby Cakes Hash Browns | 420 | |
| Nathan's Famous Jumbo Crinkle Cut French Fries! | 1330 | |
| Ore Ida Crispers! | 218 | |
| Ore Ida Diced Hash Brown Potatoes | 430 | |
| Ore Ida Fast Food Fries | 79 | |
| Ore Ida Golden Crinkles | 74 | |
| Ore Ida Golden Fries | 210 | |
| Ore Ida Golden Twirls | 20 | |
| Ore Ida Mini Tater Tots | 1170 | |

*(Continued on next page)*

| Product | Amount of Acrylamide (in parts per billion) ND = Non-detectable | Toxic Rating (Levels below 70 ppb present least risk) |
|---|---|---|
| Ore Ida Shredded Hash Brown Potatoes | 610 | 🛒 |
| Ore Ida Sweet Potato Straight Fries | 380 | 🛒 |
| Ore Ida Tater Tots | 310 | 🛒 |
| Ore Ida Waffle Fries | 120 | 🛒 |
| Ore Ida Zesties! | 67 | 🛒 |
| Red Robin Seasoned Steak Fries | 100 | 🛒 |
| Richfood French Fried Potatoes | 27 | 🛒 |
| Stahlbush Island Farms Sweet Potato (Fresh Frozen) | 50 | 🛒 |
| Wegmans Chipotle Sweet Potato Fries | 103 | 🛒 |
| Wegmans Crinkle Cut Sweet Potato Fries | 40 | 🛒 |
| Wegmans Sweet Potato Fries | 30 | 🛒 |

Jolly Time popcorn wasn't so jolly when it came to acrylamide, per the FDA's own tests. Newman's Own was, shall we say, not overly benevolent with its high acrylamide levels. Indiana Popcorn and Pop-Secret were better choices.

## Safe and Unsafe Popcorn

| Product | Amount of Acrylamide (in parts per billion) ND = Non-detectable | Toxic Rating (Levels below 70 ppb present least risk) |
|---|---|---|
| Giant Brand 94% Fat Free Butter Microwave Popcorn | 400 | 🛒 |
| Indiana Aged White Cheddar Popcorn | 40 | 🛒 |
| Jolly Time 100 Calorie Healthy Pop Kettle Microwave Popcorn | 530 | 🛒 |
| Newman's Own Light Butter Microwave Popcorn | 370 | 🛒 |
| Orville Redenbacher's Pour Over Movie Theater Butter Microwave Popcorn | 160 | 🛒 |

| Product | Amount of Acrylamide (in parts per billion) ND = Non-detectable | Toxic Rating (Levels below 70 ppb present least risk) |
|---|---|---|
| Pop-Secret Homestyle Butter Popcorn | 50 | 🛒 |
| Pop-Secret Movie Theater Butter Microwave Popcorn | 150 | 🛒 |
| Simply Balanced Popcorn Lightly Salted | 587 | 🛒 |
| Skinny Pop Popcorn | 90 | 🛒 |
| Smartfood Delight Air Popped Popcorn Sea Salt | 40 | 🛒 |

Armour and Wolf Brands have acrylamide issues kids don't need. Van Camp's Chili with Beans is the better choice. Most other soups the HLF and FDA have tested don't pose acrylamide issues and, if organic, make a safe and healthy choice. Select canned brands like Eden Foods that avoid use of the reproductive toxin bisphenol-A and related compounds.

## Safe and Unsafe Chili and Soups

| Product | Amount of Acrylamide (in parts per billion) ND = Non-detectable | Toxic Rating (Levels below 70 ppb present least risk) |
|---|---|---|
| Amy's Organic Soups Cream of Tomato Soup | ND | 🛒 |
| Applebee's Tomato Basil | 20 | 🛒 |
| Armour Chili with Beans Original | 260 | 🛒 |
| Campbell's Chunky Old Fashioned Vegetable Beef Soup | ND | 🛒 |
| Great Value Chunky Sirloin Burger Soup | ND | 🛒 |
| Health Valley Café Black Bean Soup | ND | 🛒 |
| Healthy Choice Country Vegetable Soup | 20 | 🛒 |
| Hormel Chili Chunky with Beans | 80 | 🛒 |
| Imagine Creamy Butternut Squash Soup | ND | 🛒 |
| Organic Full Circle Chicken Noodle Soup | ND | 🛒 |

*(Continued on next page)*

| Product | Amount of Acrylamide (in parts per billion) ND = Non-detectable | Toxic Rating (Levels below 70 ppb present least risk) |
|---|---|---|
| Progresso Traditional 99% Fat Free Beef Barley Soup | ND | 🛒 |
| Progresso Traditional Beef & Vegetable Soup | ND | 🛒 |
| Steak n' Shake Original Chili with Beans | 20 | 🛒 |
| Van Camp's Chili with Beans | ND | 🛒 |
| Wolf Brand Chili with Beans | 240 | 🛒 |
| Wolfgang Puck Free Range Chicken Soup with White & Wild Rice | ND | 🛒 |
| Wolfgang Puck Old Fashioned Potato Soup | 60 | 🛒 |

KC Masterpiece and Walnut Acres baked beans were the worst offenders. Walmart's Great Value is the best nonorganic choice. Black, kidney, pinto, northern, and garbanzo beans were free from acrylamide (and low in pesticides). Again, choose canned products without the bisphenol compounds.

## Safe and Unsafe Beans

| Product | Amount of Acrylamide (in parts per billion) ND = Non-detectable | Toxic Rating |
|---|---|---|
| Bush's Best Dark Red Kidney Beans | ND | 🛒 |
| Bush's Best Original Baked Beans | 20 | 🛒 |
| Bush's Best Pinto Beans | ND | 🛒 |
| Bush's Best Seasoned Recipe Black Beans | ND | 🛒 |
| Great Value Baked Beans | ND | 🛒 |
| Great Value Dark Red Kidney Beans | 10 | 🛒 |
| Great Value Pinto Beans | ND | 🛒 |
| Great Value Seasoned Black Beans | ND | 🛒 |
| KC Masterpiece Baked Beans Hickory Brown Sugar | 80 | 🛒 |
| Luck's Black Beans | ND | 🛒 |

| Product | Amount of Acrylamide (in parts per billion) ND = Non-detectable | Toxic Rating |
|---|---|---|
| Van Camp's Baked Beans Original | 27 | 🛒 |
| Walnut Acres Organic Baked Beans Vegetarian | 160 | 🛒 |
| Wild Oats Marketplace Organic Dark Red Kidney Beans | ND | 🛒 |

My kids once loved Starbucks hot chocolate. But not since learning FDA testing showed that it was loaded with acrylamide. Get Land O'Lakes Chocolate Supreme Hot Cocoa Mix, Shur, or Swiss Miss. These have the least acrylamide.

## Safe and Unsafe Hot Chocolate

| Product | Amount of Acrylamide (in parts per billion) ND = Non-detectable | Toxic Rating (Levels below 70 ppb present least risk) |
|---|---|---|
| Land O'Lakes Cocoa Classics Chocolate Supreme Hot Cocoa Mix | ND | 🛒 |
| Nestle Abuelita Authentic Mexican Chocolate Mix | 40 | 🛒 |
| Shur Fine Rich Cocoa Hot Cocoa Mix | ND | 🛒 |
| Starbucks Hot Cocoa Mix Double Chocolate | 100 | 🛒 |
| Swiss Miss Rich Chocolate Hot Cocoa Mix | 20 | 🛒 |

It's nuts—just nuts—giving kids roasted almonds. But giving them Justin's almond butters, when so many safer choices are available, is beyond nuts. Once almonds get roasted, they build up relatively high amounts of acrylamide. Isn't that what's happening to Justin's Classic Nut Butter? Yet, as our testing showed, other roasted almond nut butter brands seem to be immune from building up exorbitant amounts of acrylamide. Walmart, Kroger, MaraNatha, Whole Foods 365, and Maisie Jane's are safe choices. Roasted peanuts, cashews, walnuts, Brazil nuts, and sunflower and pumpkin seeds don't build up acrylamide like roasted almonds. Unroasted and unsalted is always healthier.

# Safe and Unsafe Nut Butters

| Product | Amount of Acrylamide (in parts per billion) ND = Non-detectable | Toxic Rating (Levels below 70 ppb present least risk) |
|---|---|---|
| 365 Everyday Value Almond Butter, Cream | 143 | ⬤ |
| Buff Bake Protein Almond Spread | 47 | 🛒 |
| Great Value Hazelnut Spread | ND | 🛒 |
| I.M. Healthy Creamy Soy Nut Butter | 13 | 🛒 |
| Jif Almond Butter Creamy | 570 | ⬤ |
| Jif Creamy Peanut Butter | 50 | 🛒 |
| Jif Natural Almond Butter Spread | 235 | ⬤ |
| Justin's Classic Nut Butter | 873 | ⬤ |
| Justin's Honey Almond Butter | 296 | ⬤ |
| Justin's Maple Almond Butter | 362 | ⬤ |
| Justin's Vanilla Almond Butter | 827 | ⬤ |
| Kroger Creamy Almond Butter | ND | 🛒 |
| Kroger Creamy Hazelnut Spread with Cocoa | ND | 🛒 |
| Maisie Jane's Smooth Almond Butter | 70 | 🛒 |
| MaraNatha Sunflower Seed Butter | ND | 🛒 |
| Noosh Almond Butter Packs Birthday Cake | ND | 🛒 |
| Nutella Hazelnut Spread with Cocoa | ND | 🛒 |
| Peter Pan 100% Natural Creamy Peanut Butter Spread | ND | 🛒 |
| RxBarNut Butter Almond Butter | 110 | ⬤ |
| Simple Truth Organic No Stir Creamy Peanut Butter | ND | 🛒 |
| Simply Balanced Almond Butter | 363 | ⬤ |
| Skippy Natural Creamy Peanut Butter Spread | 30 | 🛒 |
| SunButter Sunflower Spread | ND | 🛒 |
| Wowbutter Creamy Toasted Soy Spread | ND | 🛒 |

# Safe and Unsafe Nuts

| Product | Amount of Acrylamide (in parts per billion) ND = Non-detectable | Toxic Rating (Levels below 70 ppb present least risk) |
|---|---|---|
| Always Save Mixed Nuts | ND |  |
| Archer Farms Deluxe Roasted Mixed Nuts (Almonds, Cashews, Brazil Nuts, Hazelnuts, & Pecans) | ND |  |
| Best Choice Dry Roasted Peanuts Salted | 50 |  |
| Best Choice Honey Roasted Peanuts | 20 |  |
| Best Choice Natural Pecan Halves | ND |  |
| Blue Diamond Almonds Whole Natural | 10 |  |
| Blue Diamond Oven Roasted Almonds Sea Salt | 160 |  |
| Fisher Chef's Naturals Pecan Halves | ND |  |
| Fisher Chef's Naturals Raw Peanuts | ND |  |
| Fisher Chef's Naturals Whole Natural Almonds | ND |  |
| Great Value Almonds Roasted & Salted With Sea Salt | 100 |  |
| Great Value Almonds Whole Natural | 10 |  |
| Great Value Honey Roasted Peanuts | 20 |  |
| Great Value Unsalted Peanuts Dry Roasted | 20 |  |
| Hines Nut Co. Pecans | ND |  |
| HyVee Raw Spanish Peanuts | ND |  |
| Planters Dry Roasted Peanuts | 20 |  |
| Planters Honey Roasted Peanuts Dry Roasted | 20 |  |
| Planters Mixed Nuts (Peanuts, Cashews, Almonds, Brazil Nuts, Pecans) | ND |  |
| SunTree Raw Spanish Peanuts | ND |  |
| Superior Nut Company Honey Roasted Pecans | ND |  |
| Wonderful Roasted & Salted Almonds | 150 |  |

*(Continued on next page)*

Large black olives and prune juice are acrylamide hazards. Best Choice and Great Value, Lindsay, and Musco large black olives tested high in acrylamide and should be avoided during pregnancy. Trader Joe's, Whole Foods 365, Mario Pimiento Stuffed Spanish Olives, and Meijer Stuffed Manzanilla Olives with Minced Pimiento tested lower and are safer choices. Choose medium- and smaller-sized olives when possible. The larger-sized products tend to have more of the chemical toxin. Fig fruit is low in acrylamide. Prune juice tested high and shouldn't be consumed during pregnancy.

## Safe and Unsafe Olives and Prunes

| Product | Amount of Acrylamide (in parts per billion) ND = Non-detectable | Toxic Rating (Levels below 70 ppb present least risk) |
|---|---|---|
| 365 Everyday Value Pitted Ripe Green Olives Medium | 43 | |
| Best Choice Large Pitted Ripe Olives | 240 | |
| Clover Valley 100% Prune Juice | 170 | |
| Graber Olives | 70 | |
| Great Value 100% Prune Juice | 60 | |
| Great Value California-Style Sliced Ripe Olives | 340 | |
| Great Value Manzanilla Olives Stuffed with Minced Pimento | ND | |
| Lindsay California Ripe Pitted Olives Large | 500 | |
| Lindsay Naturals California Green Olives | 50 | |
| Mario Pimiento Stuffed Spanish Olives | ND | |
| Meijer Stuffed Manzanilla Olives with Minced Pimiento Thrown | ND | |
| Meijer Stuffed Queen Olives with Minced Pimiento Placed | 10 | |
| Musco Family Olive Co. Early California Fresh Cured Green Ripe Medium Pitted California Olives | 200 | |
| Musco Family Olive Co. Early California Medium Pitted California Ripe Olives | 290 | |

| Product | Amount of Acrylamide (in parts per billion) ND = Non-detectable | Toxic Rating (Levels below 70 ppb present least risk) |
|---|---|---|
| Musco Family Olive Co. Early California Pimento Stuffed Manzanilla Olives | 10 | 🛒 |
| Nice! Large Olives Ripe & Pitted | 450 | ⬤ |
| Roland Whole Kalamata Olives | ND | 🛒 |
| Sun-Maid California Pitted Prunes | 70 | 🛒 |
| Sunsweet Prune Juice | 200 | ⬤ |
| Trader Joe's Ripe Medium Green Pitted Olives | ND | 🛒 |

Trader Joe's Chocolately Cat Low-Fat Cookies and Old Fashioned Cinnamon Grahams were loaded with acrylamide when the HLF tested them. They were so high the HLF filed legal action against Trader Joe's for peddling tainted cookies without label warnings advising shoppers that a harmful chemical contaminated their product. (Even today, the chain's in-store so-called acrylamide "warnings" appear to me to be sorely inadequate, never specifying which products are contaminated, and probably don't comply with California law.) Nabisco Ginger Snaps are bad news, based on FDA tests. Annie's Lemon Drop cookies are a good choice. They're organic too. Pepperidge Farm is an industry leader for acrylamide safety, based on the HLF's tests.

## Safe and Unsafe Cookies, Crackers, and Granola Bars

| Product | Amount of Acrylamide (in parts per billion) ND = Non-detectable | Toxicity Rating |
|---|---|---|
| Annie's Homegrown Organic Cookie Bites, Chocolate Chips | 94 | ⬤ |
| Annie's Organic Lemon Drop Cookie Bars | ND | 🛒 |
| Annie's Organic PB&J Chewy Granola Bars | ND | 🛒 |
| Archway Homestyle Classics Crispy Gingersnap Cookies | 220 | ⬤ |
| Austin's Toasty Crackers with Peanut Butter Sandwich Crackers | 468 | ⬤ |

*(Continued on next page)*

| Product | Amount of Acrylamide (in parts per billion) ND = Non-detectable | Toxicity Rating |
|---|---|---|
| Bill Rhodes Bakery Gingerbread Cookie | 20 | 🛒 |
| Caribou Coffee Classic Milk Chocolate Chunk Cookies | 20 | 🛒 |
| Cascadian Farm Chewy Chocolate Chip Granola Bars | ND | 🛒 |
| Clif Energy Bar Chocolate Chip | 10 | 🛒 |
| Cub Fresh Ginger Cookies | 70 | 🛒 |
| Dare Breton Original | 387 | 🛒 |
| Dare Water Crackers, Cracked Pepper | ND | 🛒 |
| Essential Everyday Chewy Chocolate Chip Granola Bars | 30 | 🛒 |
| Essential Everyday Fudge Wafer Cookies | 50 | 🛒 |
| Essential Everyday Ginger Snaps | 377 | 🛒 |
| Giant Brand Crunchy Peanut Butter Granola Bar | 740 | 🛒 |
| Giant Performance Bar Peanut Butter Chocolate Chip | ND | 🛒 |
| Great Value Chewy Protein Bars Peanut Butter & Dark Chocolate | ND | 🛒 |
| Great Value Classic Chocolate Chip Cookies | 300 | 🛒 |
| Great Value Ginger Snaps | 650 | 🛒 |
| Homekist Cookies Chocolate Chip | 70 | 🛒 |
| Kashi Honey Almond Flax Chewy Granola Bars | 30 | 🛒 |
| Keebler Chips Deluxe Cookies Original | 150 | 🛒 |
| Kind Almond and Apricot Bars | ND | 🛒 |
| Lance Toasty Sandwich Crackers Peanut Butter | 189 | 🛒 |
| Larabar Fruit & Nut Food Bar Cherry Pie | 30 | 🛒 |
| Late July Organic Mini Peanut Butter Sandwich Crackers | 294 | 🛒 |

| Product | Amount of Acrylamide (in parts per billion) ND = Non-detectable | Toxicity Rating |
|---|---|---|
| Luna LemonZest Nutrition Bar | ND | 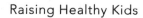 |
| Lunds & Byerlys Our Bakery Iced Ginger Cookies | 30 | |
| Lunds & Byerlys Our Bakery Sugar Cookies | ND | |
| Martha Harp's Gold Chocolate Chunk Cookies | 30 | |
| Meijer Ginger Snaps | 260 | |
| Nabisco Chips Ahoy! Chocolate Chip Cookies Original | 250 | |
| Nabisco Ginger Snaps | 1450 | |
| Nabisco Good Thins, Sweet potato | 133 | |
| Nature Valley Oats n' Honey Crunchy Granola Bars | 440 | |
| Newman's Own Ginger O's | 300 | |
| Panera Bread Toffee Nut Cookie | ND | |
| Pepperidge Farm Milano Dark Chocolate Cookies | ND | |
| Perkins Restaurant & Bakery Sugar Cookie | ND | |
| Power Bar Performance Energy Bar Chocolate | ND | |
| Power Crunch Protein Energy Bar Original | 90 | |
| Publix Bakery Cookies San Francisco Cookies | ND | |
| Pure Organic Wild Blueberry Bar | 40 | |
| Quaker Chewy S'mores Granola Bars | 20 | |
| QuestBar Protein Bar Double Chocolate Chunk | ND | |
| Safeway Kitchens Treasure Chips Original Cookies | 90 | |

*(Continued on next page)*

| Product | Amount of Acrylamide (in parts per billion) ND = Non-detectable | Toxicity Rating |
|---|---|---|
| Safeway Signature Kitchens Chocolate Chip Chewy Granola Bars | ND | 🛒 |
| ShaSha Co. Ginger Snaps Spelt | 60 | 🛒 |
| Springfield Chocolate Chip Cookies | 480 | 🛒 |
| Stauffer's Ginger Snaps | 997 | 🛒 |
| The Fresh Market Fresh Bakery Salted Caramel Cookie | 30 | 🛒 |
| ThinkThin Protein Nut Bar Chocolate Coconut Almond | ND | 🛒 |
| Trader Joe's Chocolate Chip Cookie Dunkers | ND | 🛒 |
| Trader Joe's Chocolatey Cat Low-Fat Cookies | 800 | 🛒 |
| Trader Joe's Gluten Free Ginger Snaps | 340 | 🛒 |
| Trader Joe's Old Fashioned Cinnamon Grahams | 400 | 🛒 |
| Trader Joe's Triple Ginger Snaps | 160 | 🛒 |
| Voortman Oatmeal Raisin Cookies | 40 | 🛒 |
| Wal-Mart The Bakery Signature Chocolate Chunk Cookies | 30 | 🛒 |
| Wild Oats Marketplace Organic Crunchy Peanut Butter Granola Bars | 80 | 🛒 |

Most snack companies have been responsibly improving their sourcing of raw materials and processing methods to reduce the amount of acrylamide in their products.

Justin's and General Mills use their money to bully consumers and litigate cases for years in order to keep profits pouring in at the expense of children's health. Shun them.

There are so many safer choices. You know them. You've got the power to determine the future of your kids and do the right thing. Do it!

# Welcome Home!

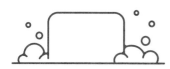

# Chapter 9

# Pretty Poisons

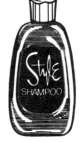

Stephanie Mero, a stylist based in Orlando, Florida, and known in social media as the "Curl Ninja" stammered. Tears streamed down her face. We spoke via Zoom during the worst days of the pandemic. I noticed her hair—it had fallen out in patches. She had shaved off the rest. Stephanie informed me she chose *not* to wear a wig because she knew others were going through the same thing and losing their hair, too. "I wanted to be strong for them," she said.

Stephanie began using Devacurl in 2016. With her dark mane's thick waves and curves, she liked that Devacurl catered to the haircare needs of "curly girls."

Initially, Stephanie's clients raved about how the Devacurl products she recommended helped them hold a curl even in the wet Florida heat. Stephanie's YouTube videos featuring Devacurl accumulated tens of thousands of views.

"But after a while, my clients began telling me their hair was thinning," Stephanie told me. "Their curls were less dense. They suffered red patches, irritation, and scalp infections. Hair began falling out of my scalp, too."

Clients mentioned irregular and absent periods, miscarriages, and difficulty getting pregnant, Stephanie said.

Stephanie had to admit she was suffering the same symptoms and never connected them to her haircare products. "But now I could see everything began happening around the same time; it took my own hair falling out to make it all real. . . ."

Stephanie initiated a call to Devacurl and spoke with the company's in-house stylist.

"They just wanted me to feel heard and hoped that would be enough to make me go away," Stephanie recounted. "Their in-house stylist kept telling me how sorry she was for my experience with their products. I wanted to share what my clients were experiencing, I told her. Something bad to their health was happening. Devacurl needed to know: my clients were getting hurt. But she told me they only wanted to hear about my own personal experience and not theirs. It was demeaning and humiliating. I tried to explain being a stylist herself, she would understand how important it was for me to convey their complaints. After all, I recommended the products to them, and now they were getting sick, but she wouldn't allow me to share what was happening to them."

Devacurl did toss her clients a bone and offered to extend the return window just for them, Stephanie said.

"Wasn't that sweet?" I retorted.

"I wanted to get out of there as fast as possible," Stephanie observed. "It was uncomfortable."

I met Stephanie when she was sharing her experience for *Not So Pretty*, the Max documentary that uncovers the beauty industry's dirty secrets. My task with Stephanie was to help her figure out which ingredients or contaminants in the products were causing so much health mayhem with her clients, herself, and thousands of other Devacurl users—while the crew filmed what was sometimes an emotionally charged conversation.

Stephanie and her partner, who also worked in the beauty industry, wanted to start a family. They didn't want to quit their jobs. But now she was thinking she might have to give up what she loved or else lose the last shreds of health that remained in her fatigued, worn-out body.

A several-hour meeting and filming ensued. Stephanie noted the synthetic fragrances used in the products were a source of hidden chemical toxins. In addition, at the time her clients began reporting their injuries, Devacurl undertook a significant change to its plastic packaging "resulting in a chemical reaction that caused the products to turn brown on the bottom." There is a great deal of credence to what Stephanie observed. After all, fragrance is a source of parabens, musk ketone, aldehydes, phthalates, benzophenone, and other toxic chemicals. She also witnessed and documented the change in the packaging and appearance of the products. Once I began looking at the product labels themselves, something else quite obvious stood out to me, and it was kind of horrible, especially for persons of color and those with curly or kinky hair. The six Devacurl products Stephanie and her clients were using the most were loaded with a family of chemicals frequently added to haircare formulas designed for those with curls. The chemicals are technically known as quaternium ammonium compounds. Beauty professionals call them "quats." There are hundreds of them, many so similar that upon introduction into commercial use for the haircare market, they are given only numbers for names, such as quaternium-15 (17, 87, or 91). They're cheap. They work well.

We all know how difficult it can be to comb out a head full of hair after shampooing when your strands are filled with static electricity and stuck together. Quat-based conditioners soften, condition, and detangle hair fibers by taking away the static electricity. The quats cover the scaly, rough surfaces of hair strands to make them slick and slippery. They repel water, which is why curls last longer. Plus, they're difficult to wash out, so their effects last. Sounds great, doesn't it? The industry loves them. It's a two-for-one deal. Their customers get better curls, and manufacturers save on added preservatives since the quats kill almost every microorganism they come in contact with.

The trouble is, ever since the pandemic, we've been on quat overload.[1] That's because the same quats the beauty industry is asking women of color and others with curls or kinky hair to use daily are the main disinfectant ingredient in sanitary hand wipes, bathroom cleaners, and Lysol spray disinfectant. The quats have their place—they're valuable in our fight against pathogens, including the coronavirus, but they hardly belong on anybody's scalp or in women's wombs.

The personal-care and cosmetic industry has long been regulated by fewer than two pages of federal law hidden away among the hundreds that make up the 1938 US Food, Drug, and Cosmetic Act.

The Food and Drug Administration's (FDA) Office of Colors and Cosmetics has an annual budget of eight million dollars and fewer than thirty employees.[2]

The US cosmetic industry has revenues north of seventy billion dollars annually and employs more than one million persons including stylists, manicurists, cosmetologists, and shop workers.[3, 4]

The law allows the industry to self-regulate by funding its own Cosmetic Ingredient Review panels comprising scientists whose salaries are covered by those they are there to oversee. No one represents the public interest on any CIR panel, including the one that reviewed the safety of quats.[5]

What could possibly go wrong?

In fact, the beauty industry has been keeping a dirty little secret about the quats: a 2014 study on their reproductive toxicity that never made it to even the references of any industry-funded published opinion on the safety of these compounds.[6]

That year, Virginia Tech researchers, writing in *Reproductive Toxicology*, reported an unusual case of mass infertility among their mice populations at the university's Biomedical Lab.[7] They observed decreased reproductive performance in laboratory mice coincided with the introduction of a disinfectant containing quats. Breeding pairs exposed for six months to the disinfectant just as it was sprayed during normal use exhibited noticeable decreases in fertility and fecundity, increased time to first litter, longer pregnancy intervals, and fewer pups and pregnancies, the investigators wrote. Fetal deaths during pregnancy increased.

Follow-up research showed male mice exposed to quats had lower sperm concentrations with decreased motility. Another study found increased rates of neural tube defects in the offspring of mice exposed to quats.[8, 9]

In 2021, scientists began measuring the quats in human blood for the first time and found they harm mitochondria (the cells' energy factories), alter cholesterol metabolism, and increase inflammation.[10]

The quats were effectively outlawed in Europe almost immediately following the Virginia Tech study.[11, 12] Here in America, the CIR panel instead recommended multiple quats could be used in products.[13]

Devacurl literally doubled down on their use. They appeared to have overloaded their product formulas with multiple quats to provide the styling effect their marketers desired.

Yet, unsuspecting women and men (particularly African Americans and other persons of color) who use such products won't know their infertility is being caused by haircare products. This is especially relevant to the health of African American women, who use more of them than white females.[14]

"Black women are overexposed and under-protected from toxic chemicals," said Janette Robinson Flint, executive director of Black Women for Wellness, a Los Angeles-based social services organization.

The Centers for Disease Control and Prevention has found Black women experience earlier puberty and higher rates of hormone-related health conditions, such as uterine fibroids, infertility, breast cancer, and preterm births, than white females.[15, 16]

Could beauty products be part of the problem? African American women were also found in a study to be at higher risk for breast cancer from using chemical hair straighteners.[17] Silent Spring Institute, a breast cancer prevention nonprofit organization based in Newton, Massachusetts, examined eighteen different products geared toward Black women. These included hot oil treatments, anti-frizz hair polishes, leave-in conditioners, root stimulators, scalp lotions, and relaxers.[18] More than 70 percent of the tested products were rich in endocrine-disrupting chemicals.

Stacy Malkan, founder of the Safe Cosmetics Campaign and author of *Not Just a Pretty Face: The Ugly Side of the Beauty Industry*, puts it all together. "It isn't just one chemical in one product. It's the totality."

Calling herself a "former makeup addict," Stacy itemized the daily beauty routine she religiously performed as a high school cheerleader. From lotion to foundation to hair spray, nineteen products total, Stacy looked up each one in the Environmental Working Group's (EWG) comprehensive Skin Deep ingredient database available at www.ewg.org/skindeep/.

"I was exposing myself to two hundred thirty chemicals every day before I even got on the bus for school," she said. "And it was all legal."

## Pretty Poisons—A Family Protection Plan

Thankfully, the beauty market, under consumer pressure, is moving in a safer, healthier, truly caring direction. These safe, plant-based ingredients emulate quats without toxicity:

- **AminoSensyl HC**, an amino acid conditioning agent, adds rich texture, softens, smoothens, and offers styling propertics much like any other of the quat compounds.
- **ProCondition Sativa**, derived from *Cannabis* seed oil, is comparable in performance to cetrimonium chloride.
- **ProCondition 22**, derived from veggies such as broccoli and other members of the brassica family, emulates behentrimonium chloride.

By the way, quats are listed on the label. Just look for the "i-u-m" at the end of the name, as in behentrimonium or cetrimonium chloride, which is a tell-tale sign.

## Safe Curls, Healthy Girls

The Campaign for Safe Cosmetics and Breast Cancer Prevention Partners (BCPP) have been busily networking with Black beauty entrepreneurs whose companies are at the forefront in developing and marketing safe and healthy hair and skin care products as part of a much-needed Top Non-Toxic Black-Owned Beauty Brands database. The campaign deserves praise for putting together this vital directory and applying a zero-tolerance standard to ensure the brands represent the ultimate in safe use for the African American and ethnic hair-care communities. Visit safecosmetics.org/black-beauty-project/ to access this very useful database.

I've evaluated the major haircare brands in the chart below to make your shopping choices quick and easy. Safe brands generally use clean ingredients throughout their product line. Unsafe ones usually offer products with consistently dirty ingredients.

### Safe and Unsafe Haircare Product Brands

🛒 = Safe, none, or least risk

🛒 = Dangerous

| Product | Reproductive and Developmental Risk | Cancer Risk |
| --- | --- | --- |
| Annemarie Börlind | 🛒 | 🛒 |
| Aussie Miracles Curls | 🛒 | 🛒 |
| Avalon Organics | 🛒 | 🛒 |
| Aveeno | 🛒 | 🛒 |
| Burt's Bees | 🛒 | 🛒 |
| Cantu | 🛒 | 🛒 |
| Carol's Daughter | 🛒 | 🛒 |
| Curly Kids | 🛒 | 🛒 |
| Everyone 3-in-1 Kids Soap, Body Wash, Bubble Bath, Shampoo | 🛒 | 🛒 |
| Head & Shoulders | 🛒 | 🛒 |
| Light Mountain Natural Hair Color | 🛒 | 🛒 |

| Product | Reproductive and Developmental Risk | Cancer Risk |
|---|:---:|:---:|
| Maui Moisture | 🛒 (filled) | 🛒 (filled) |
| Miss Jessie's Multicultural Curls | 🛒 (filled) | 🛒 (filled) |
| Mixed Chicks | 🛒 (filled) | 🛒 (filled) |
| Mustela Baby Gentle Cleansing Gel - Baby Hair & Body Wash | 🛒 (outline) | 🛒 (outline) |
| Pacifica | 🛒 (outline) | 🛒 (outline) |
| Pantene | 🛒 (filled) | 🛒 (filled) |
| Prose | 🛒 (outline) | 🛒 (outline) |
| Puracy Shampoo & Body Wash for Children | 🛒 (outline) | 🛒 (outline) |
| Pureology | 🛒 (filled) | 🛒 (filled) |
| SheaMoisture | 🛒 (outline) | 🛒 (outline) |
| Stephanie Mero | 🛒 (outline) | 🛒 (outline) |
| The Honest Company | 🛒 (outline) | 🛒 (outline) |
| TRESemmé | 🛒 (filled) | 🛒 (filled) |
| Uncle Funky's Daughter Curly Magic | 🛒 (outline) | 🛒 (outline) |

Quats aren't the only toxic threat from beauty products.

Parabens are preservatives with estrogenic effects. Their presence in high amounts in cancerous breast tumors is a troubling finding.[19, 20] They're used in skin lotions and deodorants. Fortunately, at least for informed shoppers who know to look, their presence is listed on product labels, and they can be largely avoided.

A more troubling toxicity issue is the everywhere-yet-hidden presence of phthalates, which are never listed on labels. Phthalates are microplastics that fix fragrances into products with their heavy molecular weight, make them cling to your skin, and add thickness to sprays and lotions. They also act like plastic nanoparticles in the brain and testes and block the actions of testosterone, heighten the actions of estrogen, or do both, depending on which one is being studied and their endless combinations.

I tested English Leather cologne my son, Spenser, brought home. It was loaded with phthalates, but none were listed.[21] The Canoe fragrance my daughter bought was loaded, too.[22] Phthalates are everywhere in cosmetics.

Phthalate-exposed kids lose IQ points, cognitive power, and language skills.[23] They have less working cortical brain tissue just like the kids with high pesticide exposures in the CHAMACOS study.[24] Their fertility is impaired and sexual anatomy altered toward the feminine.[25] They exhibit feminized play behavior.[26, 27, 28] In girls, exposures lead to hyperfeminization or masculinization of behavior, polycystic ovary disease, and endometriosis.[29, 30, 31] The amounts causing toxic effects in these studies are drawn from the bodily fluids of normal, everyday moms and children.[32] That's why reducing your exposure is of paramount importance.

Despite the fact that phthalates have been banned for children's toys and pacifiers, no such limits exist for beauty and personal-care products even though they are readily absorbed through the skin of newborns and found in products used daily during vulnerable periods of brain growth.

Johnson & Johnson's offers so-called no-phthalate baby products. The company widely advertises theirs are free of phthalates. But, in fact, their products are loaded with them, including with some of the most toxic, heavily studied phthalates known to science, according to testing commissioned by the Healthy Living Foundation (HLF).

The HLF's testing, performed at multiple independent laboratories, identified seventeen Johnson's baby products with a variety of phthalates—despite the company's claims.

Some twenty-three million Americans used Johnson's Baby Lotion in 2020, according to Statista.com.[33] Almost twenty-four million used the baby shampoo. Johnson & Johnson's share of the baby-care market worldwide was expected to be just under 18 percent in 2021, notes Statista.[34]

Very often, a baby's first bath at the hospital and upon arriving home is with Johnson's. In the days and months following birth, your baby's fragile brain is developing at the same rate or faster than when they were in the womb. Coding errors become multiplied.

The risk of damaged gene function "is higher when the exposure occurs during periods of increased vulnerability, such as prenatal, perinatal, and early postnatal life," researchers wrote.[35]

This time period, known as the brain growth spurt, starts during the third trimester of pregnancy through the first two years of life.

The HLF sued Johnson & Johnson in the Superior Court for the District of Columbia for violations of the Consumer Procedures Protection Act. As this is being written, the case was remanded to federal court. Because legal cases can move slowly, here are the seventeen Johnson's formulas that tested positive for phthalates:

1. Baby Bar Soap
2. Cologne
3. Creamy Oil with Aloe & Vitamin E
4. Lotion
5. Baby Shampoo
6. Bedtime Baby Lotion
7. Bedtime Baby Bubble Bath
8. Cotton Touch Newborn Face & Body Lotion
9. Cotton Touch Newborn Wash & Shampoo
10. Head-to-Toe Lotion
11. Head-to-Toe Baby Wash and Shampoo
12. Head-to-Toe Baby Cleansing Cloths
13. Lavender Powder
14. Skin Nourish Vanilla Oat Wash
15. Strengthening Conditioner
16. Strengthening Shampoo
17. Soothing Vapor Bath

So, if you do a beauty intervention, will it actually work and reduce kids' toxic exposures? Once again, the Salinas CHAMACOS youth succinctly and definitively have answered this question. They teamed up with Dr. Kim Harley, a reproductive epidemiologist at UC Berkeley, to recruit one hundred Latina girls, ages fourteen to eighteen, as participants in the Health and Environmental Research in Make-up of Salinas Adolescents (HERMOSA) intervention.[36] (*Hermosa* in Spanish means "pretty.")

The youths recruited participants through social media, word of mouth, and personal networks. The teenaged girls in the study received one hundred dollars in coupons for their participation plus replacement personal-care products with clean ingredients. Levels of toxic chemicals in their urine were measured before and after the three-day beauty-product intervention.

Once the teens began using the safer beauty products, within only three days, concentrations of phthalates decreased by 27 percent. Methyl and propyl paraben concentrations decreased by 44 and 45 percent, respectively. Concentrations of triclosan (a fake estrogen that causes fetal malformations and miscarriages) and benzophenone (toxic to breast cells) each decreased by 36 percent.[37]

Each of these chemicals is a fake estrogen or anti-androgen. The study participants were on their way to not only greater personal health but, should they choose, complication-free pregnancies, and healthier, brighter children. It's simple, meaningful, and works.

Do a beauty intervention. Present your children with safe beauty products. Buy them for them. They're learning while you're protecting them.

## Ditch Dioxane

In 2010, I sued Procter & Gamble and other brands when our testing found high levels of dioxane, a male breast carcinogen, in baby bubble bath, body wash, and shampoos such as Herbal Essences and Pantene.[38, 39] The court-approved consent judgment required the personal-care product company to either label their products for the presence of dioxane or significantly reduce its presence.[40] Today, when tested, Herbal Essences and Pantene products have reduced dioxane levels by 90 percent to avoid having to put warnings on their product labels. I prefer zero tolerance, of course. Nonetheless, this victory made internet headlines and led other brands to reformulate their products. But many companies haven't gotten the message. That's why parents must remain vigilant.

In this case, reading product labels will help spill the beans. Avoid products listing laureth, myreth, polyethylene glycol (PEG), ceteareth, glycereth, phenoxyethanol, polysorbate, and nonoxynol compounds, and any other label ingredients with eth in their name.

These ingredients are alcohol ethoxylates, which become contaminated with dioxane during their manufacture. They're found in shampoos, body washes, bubble baths, liquid hand soaps, and lotions. Sadly, dioxane is also being frequently found in our nation's public drinking water supplies. Please discard products containing such troubling compounds.

Choose kid-safe bubble baths, shampoos, and body washes with these safe ingredients:

- cocamidopropyl hydroxysultaine
- coco glucoside
- decyl glucoside
- disodium cocoyl glutamate
- hydroxypropyl sulfonate
- lauryl glucoside
- sodium cocoyl hydrolyzed soy protein

I've reviewed ingredient labels for the major brands of bubble bath, washes, and shampoos to show you which are safe and unsafe.

## Safe and Unsafe Kids' Body Washes, Bubble Baths, and Shampoos

| 🛒 = Safe, none, or least risk | | |
|---|---|---|
| 🛒 = Dangerous | | |

| Product | Reproductive and Developmental Risk | Cancer Risk |
|---|---|---|
| Amazon Basics Baby Shampoo, Lavender & Chamomile Scented | 🛒 | 🛒 |
| Aveeno Baby Sensitive Skin Bubble Bath with Oat Extract | 🛒 | 🛒 |
| Babo Botanicals Moisturizing Plant-Based 2-in-1 Bubble Bath & Wash | 🛒 | 🛒 |
| Baby Bum Bubble Bath | 🛒 | 🛒 |
| Baby Dove Sensitive Skin Care Baby Wash for Baby Bath | 🛒 | 🛒 |
| Baby Jolie Baby 2-in-1 Hair and Body Wash | 🛒 | 🛒 |
| Baby Magic Gentle Hair & Body Wash Oil | 🛒 | 🛒 |
| Baby Shark Body Wash and Shampoo | 🛒 | 🛒 |

*(Continued on next page)*

Raising Healthy Kids

| Product | Reproductive and Developmental Risk | Cancer Risk |
| --- | --- | --- |
| Babyganics Bubble Bath, Fragrance Free | 🛒 | 🛒 |
| Babyology All-Natural Baby Wash and Shampoo | 🛒 | 🛒 |
| Burt's Bees Baby Bee Bubble Bath | ⛟ | ⛟ |
| California Baby | 🛒 | 🛒 |
| CeraVe Baby Wash & Shampoo 2-in-1 Tear-Free Baby Wash for Baby Skin & Hair | 🛒 | 🛒 |
| Cetaphil Baby Wash & Shampoo with Organic Calendula | ⛟ | ⛟ |
| Dial Kids 3 in 1 Body+Hair+Bubble Bath | ⛟ | ⛟ |
| Everyone 3-in-1 Kids Soap, Body Wash, Bubble Bath, Shampoo | 🛒 | 🛒 |
| Finding Nemo Bath | ⛟ | ⛟ |
| The Honest Company | 🛒 | 🛒 |
| Johnson's | ⛟ | ⛟ |
| Mr. Bubble Kids Extra Gentle 4-in-1 Body Wash, Shampoo, Conditioner | ⛟ | ⛟ |
| Mustela Baby Gentle Cleansing Gel—Baby Hair & Body Wash | 🛒 | 🛒 |
| Paw Patrol Shampoo | ⛟ | ⛟ |
| Puracy Shampoo & Body Wash for Children | 🛒 | 🛒 |
| SheaMoisture Baby Wash & Shampoo for All Skin Types Raw Shea, Chamomile & Argan Oil Baby Wash and Shampoo | 🛒 | 🛒 |
| The Honest Company Foaming Bubble Bath | 🛒 | 🛒 |
| TruKid Bubble Podz Bubble Bath | 🛒 | 🛒 |
| Vivvi & Bloom Gentle 2-in-1 Baby Wash & Shampoo Cleansing Gel | 🛒 | 🛒 |

## Safer Salons

Stay away from unsafe salons. It's very dangerous for adults, more so for your embryo or fetus, when the salon management allows toxic fumes to permeate the workplace. Be sure your favorite places follow these guidelines from the California Healthy Nail Salon Collaborative:[41]

1. Nail polishes must be without the Big 3: phthalates, toluene, and formaldehyde.
2. All nail polish removers should be free from ethyl or butyl acetate.
3. Thinners must eliminate toluene and methyl ethyl ketone.
4. Ensures ventilation is fierce.
5. Nails are done in a separate area.
6. Customers cannot bring in their own products unless the management says they meet least-toxic standards.
7. Confirms disinfectant products are free from quats and triclosan.[42]

## Keep It Simple

A super clean beauty product keeps its ingredients simple. Dr. Hauschka, Logona, Weleda, Avalon, Dr. Bronner's, Burt's Bees, Botanical Rush, Honest Company, MyVeg, Simply Organic, and Credobeauty.com are among the growing number of safe brands that offer clean lines, according to my review of their label ingredients.

When you see a brand rated as safe, it will be usually the case throughout their product line. Same for the bad ones, which are most often systemically dirty.

### Safe and Unsafe Beauty Brands

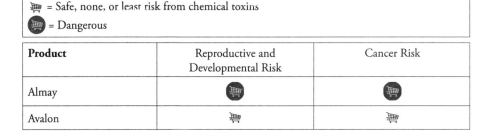

| Product | Reproductive and Developmental Risk | Cancer Risk |
|---|---|---|
| Almay | 🛒 | 🛒 |
| Avalon | 🛒 | 🛒 |

*(Continued on next page)*

| Product | Reproductive and Developmental Risk | Cancer Risk |
|---|---|---|
| Aveeno | 🛒 | 🛒 |
| Beefriendly | 🛒 | 🛒 |
| Botanical Rush | 🛒 | 🛒 |
| Burt's Bees | 🛒 | 🛒 |
| Cetaphil | ●🛒 | ●🛒 |
| Chanel | ●🛒 | ●🛒 |
| Covergirl | ●🛒 | ●🛒 |
| Curél | ●🛒 | ●🛒 |
| Dior | ●🛒 | ●🛒 |
| Dr. Hauschka | 🛒 | 🛒 |
| e.l.f. | ●🛒 | ●🛒 |
| elta md | ●🛒 | ●🛒 |
| Eminence Organic Skincare | 🛒 | 🛒 |
| Gold Bond | ●🛒 | ●🛒 |
| Jergens | ●🛒 | ●🛒 |
| Kleem Organics | 🛒 | 🛒 |
| L'Oreal | ●🛒 | ●🛒 |
| Lancôme | ●🛒 | ●🛒 |
| Logona | 🛒 | 🛒 |
| Lubriderm | ●🛒 | ●🛒 |
| Luminess | ●🛒 | ●🛒 |
| MAC | ●🛒 | ●🛒 |
| Maybelline | ●🛒 | ●🛒 |

| Product | Reproductive and Developmental Risk | Cancer Risk |
|---|---|---|
| MyVeg | 🛒 (outline) | 🛒 (outline) |
| Neutrogena | 🛒 (filled) | 🛒 (filled) |
| Nivea | 🛒 (outline) | 🛒 (outline) |
| NYX | 🛒 (filled) | 🛒 (filled) |
| OGX | 🛒 (filled) | 🛒 (filled) |
| Olay | 🛒 (filled) | 🛒 (filled) |
| Remedial Naturals | 🛒 (filled) | 🛒 (filled) |
| Revbloom | 🛒 (outline) | 🛒 (outline) |
| Revlon | 🛒 (filled) | 🛒 (filled) |
| Secret | 🛒 (filled) | 🛒 (filled) |
| Simply Organic | 🛒 (outline) | 🛒 (outline) |
| SNG Organics | 🛒 (outline) | 🛒 (outline) |
| Solimo | 🛒 (filled) | 🛒 (filled) |
| Suave | 🛒 (filled) | 🛒 (filled) |
| The Honest Company | 🛒 (outline) | 🛒 (outline) |
| US Organic | 🛒 (outline) | 🛒 (outline) |
| Vaseline | 🛒 (filled) | 🛒 (filled) |
| Weleda | 🛒 (outline) | 🛒 (outline) |

Stephanie's willingness to share some of the most painful moments of her life on her social media, particularly on Facebook where the Devacurl user group she formed has more than sixty thousand members, changed the lives of thousands of persons. She educated Devacurl users who might have never connected their hair loss, scalp burns, and reproductive health issues to the haircare products they were using. She made it possible for the users to connect with each other online and share their stories.

"It's a very powerful group," Stephanie says proudly.

The Facebook forum she created was an undeniable force in the court-approved class-action settlement thousands of Devacurl users reached with the company in January 2022, although no amount of money can make up for anybody's loss of health.[43]

For Stephanie, detox involved going plastic free and seeking formulas with short ingredient lists where she could pronounce all of the names and didn't need an encyclopedia of hazardous chemicals to identify which were safe and unsafe. She especially liked a few of the European brands packaged in glass. "Plant-based with simple ingredient lists whenever possible," she said. "Always fragrance free."

One of her favorites? "It's called MyVeg," she told me. (We went over the ingredients, and they were super clean.)

MyVeg is featured online at Curlpromise.com, the website Stephanie created to share her clean beauty product discoveries (including her own newly introduced haircare line, branded with her name, Stephanie Mero).

"What mattered the most was changing my entire diet and consumer purchase behavior to avoid the toxins that might have played a part in my poisoning—petrochemicals, synthetic fragrances, and formaldehyde releasers," Stephanie told me. "It's impossible to entirely avoid these things but making an active effort definitely helps a lot. There's nothing smarter you could do when purchasing beauty products than to avoid these chemicals.

"After about a year of being plastic and fragrance free, I decided I wanted to have a baby. I got pregnant right away and had a sickness-free pregnancy with no complications and a two-hour natural labor and birth. Unheard of. I believe my avoidance of chemical toxins helped a lot. Now I'm raising my ten-month-old son."

I recently saw the Curl Ninja's latest Instagram post.

Stephanie's thick, wavy curly strands were back. Her son Maximillian's curls were just beginning to show.

We're making a difference. Safe beauty advocates enjoyed the satisfaction of knowing their voices and commitment to voting, both at the ballot box and with their shopping dollars, were heard, loud and clear, by our nation's elected leaders when President Joseph R. Biden signed the "Modernization of Cosmetic Regulation Act of 2022" into law on December 29 of that year.[44]

The new law requires increased FDA oversight of cosmetics and the ingredients in them.[45] It establishes a process similar to those for other federally regulated products that ensures the cosmetic manufacturers register their products with the government and provide assurances they are safe.

The US Health and Human Services secretary would be able to suspend a cosmetic entity's registration if there is a reasonable probability a product is causing seriously adverse health effects or death. This gives activists and non-governmental organizations like EWG, the HLF, and Safe Cosmetics Campaign, a wide lane to petition the government, which is a Constitutional right.

Some of the most important labeling provisions, such as for fragrance allergens, however, won't go into effect for years. Nothing in the newly passed law requires companies to disclose their use of phthalates.

Persons of childbearing age, pregnant women, and parents can't wait for the law to catch up to their health needs now. Fortunately, in another universe, far away from Estee Lauder, Maybelline, Lancome, and NYX—all of which HLF testing showed contain undisclosed reproductive toxins—safe beauty products abound.

Now, you know how to say no but also *yes* to some of the most important shopping choices a parent can make for themselves and their offspring. The healthy values we affirm with our beauty-product choices are making sure that our voices are heard—bold and loud—in the nation's capitol. You win. Your kids win. We win.

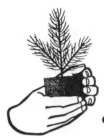

# Chapter 10
## "Believe the Moms!"

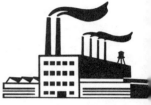

Mooresville, in Iredell County, North Carolina, is the gateway to Lake Norman. Lined by homes, waters filled with bass, bluegill, catfish, and crappie, the state's vast inland sea covers more than five hundred miles. Just outside the Charlotte metro region, the Mooresville area seemed the perfect place to raise a young family in 2008. Susan and David Wind had the opportunity to move there from their home in Coral Springs, Florida, to start new jobs. They went to Charlotte often for on-site meetings involved with their freelance tech work. They liked the mountains in the distance and living amid a forested and watery dreamscape.

"We found a real estate agent who took us all over Lake Norman, and we just fell in love," Susan told me as she began her story.

They could go boating in and out of all the little fingers and inlets or hiking along the wooded shore.

"Mommy, what's that cloud maker?" Brendan, her son, then six, asked during their early days there, strolling down the street, learning about their new community. Susan pushed her stroller with her two-year-old daughter Lexi. David and Susan's older daughter, Taylor, then seven, walked alongside their mom. The kids had a lot of questions about where they lived.

"I told them it was a steam station, but I did not know much more." Susan recalled the cool lake breeze blowing through Taylor's brown strands of hair that touched her shoulders.

"And what's that big dome, Mommy?" Taylor had asked, snuggling in close to her mother's side as they walked along under the poplars and cottonwoods. The big dome made from steel-reinforced concrete loomed outside and across the lake.

"It was to the south of where we lived and in my backyard practically," Susan informed me. "I found out the 'cloud maker' was a coal-ash burning steam station. The big dome was the McGuire nuclear plant. These were not things the real estate agent mentioned. When we would ask people, they would say our community must be safe or they would not live here."

When Taylor was a teen, she experienced different ongoing health issues. Taylor's symptoms included migraines, weight fluctuations, night sweats, and stomach pains.

"I would take her to the doctor, and she would just say, 'Mom, this is a teenager. They're hormonal at this age.'"

Two years into Taylor's symptoms, she developed a pea-sized lump on the side of her neck.

Susan took Taylor back to the doctor to have the lump checked.

"It's a swollen gland, Mom," the doctor said in a tone that Susan felt was passive-aggressive, meant to educate the mother of her patient about who knew better. "You folks have allergies, right?"

"I thought to myself, yes, we all have allergies, but none of us have ever had a small hard lump protrude out of our necks," Susan said. "In the meantime, I had been hearing for a few years about a lot of cancers in the neighborhood. My mother told me she never met so many people with cancer in her life until she moved here to be near."

It was May 2017. Susan went to see her dentist. The hygienist talked about a college tour with her daughter.

"The dental hygienist then tells me how her daughter dropped out of school because she got lymphoma, a cancer. It started with a lump on her neck."

Susan went cold.

"As soon as I got home, I called my doctor and asked her to see my daughter immediately."

After scans, tests, and biopsies, seven weeks later, on June 28, 2017, Susan received her child's diagnosis.

"My sixteen-year-old daughter had papillary thyroid cancer that had spread throughout her neck."

Susan shared Taylor's story via social media, and the floodgates opened.

"People from all over town started contacting me when they heard the news," Susan recounted. "What became more alarming was two neighbors down the street had thyroid cancer too, along with a woman who had moved out a couple years prior. This was three, and Taylor made the fourth. I also had many mothers contact me and found out a lot of girls as young as nine years old in my immediate area had thyroid cancer. I contacted our new doctors who would be treating our daughter to find out if this was normal (the numbers I collected had started to add up). They said NO! Something is not right. The questions started to make my head spin. Was this area safe? Was my home safe? Could it be the water? Air? What was happening here? I pleaded with experts to find out if someone could help me to start an environmental study and answer these questions with confidence."

Six months later, while taking care of a sick teenager, working full time, and managing her family, Susan went online to start a fundraiser to get the study started. She raised $109,000.

"The stories were heartbreaking and people just knew something was not right," Susan said. "House after house, people had cancers. The dogs and cats had cancer. People who lived in a home had cancer and then moved out, and the new tenants got cancer there years later. It was so much. I started collecting all of their data, too. What was going on? I had parents contact me one by one. Their teenagers attended our local high school (some of them were different years than my daughter). The list kept growing (thyroid, leukemia, lymphomas, testicular, brain, and lung cancers). The town south of us on the lake, near the nuclear plant, had an ocular melanoma cancer cluster (which the state again tried to downplay). The rarest cancers were hitting young girls in that area, which was not normal.

"Friends told me to contact local government officials. This is how it starts. You go through the locals, then state, and federal officials. This is an entirely broken system unable to protect us and completely full of BS, to be brutally honest.

"The first meeting at a coffee shop involved North Carolina State Senator Vicki Sawyer, John Fraley, who was then a member of the North Carolina House of Representatives, and Miles Atkins, the mayor of Mooresville. I shared my findings with them and showed them a hand-drawn map of where all of these cancers were popping up, and I asked them to help. Representative Fraley said, 'Do you think this is linked to Duke Energy and the coal ash?' His second question was, 'Has anyone from the utility company tried to contact you? Scare you?' I am just thinking to myself: what is coal ash, and why would someone from the utility company try to intimidate me? And what does he know, and why is he asking me these questions?

"I had been trying to get state health records of the incidence of thyroid and other cancers for months. I noticed the data were so outdated, the statistics were already three to four years old; they did not even have many cancers listed on their website. When I would ask questions, I got marginal answers. I learned throughout this 'environmental advocacy' when you ask questions, hard questions, you get total hostility in return, as if you shouldn't ask questions but just shut up, get over your kid's sickness, and be thankful you live in such a great county, state, and country and all the crap they throw at you when you're pressing them because your daughter is sick. The chemist I commissioned had to have a bunch of meetings with the North Carolina health department folks as well in order to obtain the most current data and determine if we had a cluster. Finally we get an email. The zip code I lived in had a thyroid cancer cluster."

In *NC Policy Watch*, journalist Lisa Sorg wrote: "The state's Central Cancer Registry statistics show that for the past twenty-two years, Iredell County has reported statistically higher incidences of thyroid cancer than the state average—even double or three times greater."[1]

In October 2018, with the historically heavy regional rains, sludge-like soil started to bubble up beside Taylor's high school. It was frightening to both of them and made them feel like they were taking part in a horror film.

"I contacted another chemist from Duke University who worked closely with the one I commissioned," Susan said. "He was an expert on coal ash. I educated myself real fast and learned the only people who said it was safe were utility companies and their paid scientists. My stomach sank. I had moved to a town that used toxic coal ash to landscape flower beds, build homes, fill parks and schools, pave roads, and that lies under shopping centers. This was not safe. It was not safe in the soil, water, or air. We were being poisoned."

Susan started to go through the state Department of Environmental Quality online records. This was the state agency supposed to "regulate" the environment, she thought. Instead, she found documents that provided evidence some forty-three thousand tons of coal ash had been dumped (abandoned) in 2001 next to the high school where the gray sludge bubbled to the surface. Iredell County Board of Commissioner member James Mallory, with whom she also met (although he later appeared "dishonest" when she learned more about what he never told her at their first meeting), "had actually signed off on the dirt in 2001," she later discovered. "He forgot to mention that to me when we had our initial meeting. Now I had an actual record of this dirt and too many kids with cancer.

The list is still climbing as kids who have graduated, moved on, and are in their twenties, contact me."[2, 3]

Coal ash is not only a carcinogen; it synergizes and magnifies the toxic effects of radiation. The combination is far more toxic than either alone. Coal ash is rich in microelements such as chromium, manganese, and strontium. Iodine-131, the kind of radiation released from a nuclear plant, causes thyroid cancer.[4] A 2021 article in the journal *Biometals* found these heavy metals synergize thyroid cancers, making them even more invasive.[5, 6, 7] Thus, the combination of nuclear radiation and coal ash's heavy metals is an even more deadly poison to the children of Mooresville. Most people there don't even know they should be protecting their families from these hazards that Susan unearthed.

"People need to know the truth and become educated on what is going on not only in Mooresville but America," Susan continued angrily. "All pollutants should be disclosed to everyone so they can make a choice. I had no choice. I never knew about the coal ash. If I did, I would never have moved to Mooresville and maybe I could have spared my daughter from the cancer she has been dealing with since June 2017.

"The system is broken," she said. "More and more kids are getting cancer. Whether it's poly- and perfluorylalkyl substances (PFAS), coal ash, or the chemicals used to manufacture micro-plastics, stories like mine are happening to children and families in real time all over the country. Believe the moms!"

## "Believe the Moms!"—A Family Protection Plan

Susan tells people, "Before you move anywhere, do your research. Look up the nearest chemical, power, and nuclear plants, paper mills, Superfund sites, and brownfields [a tract of polluted, abandoned land developed for industrial purposes]. Do searches to find out everything you can about the environmental issues of your town or community to see if parents like me brought these issues to the forefront."

Just what are the questions we should be asking? Here's a comprehensive list to complete a toxic inventory of your own community:

1. **Do I live in a pollution hot zone?** Enter "The Most Detailed Map of Cancer-Causing Industrial Air Pollution in the US" into your favorite search engine to link with *Propublica's* interactive chart that shows local toxic sites. Use your present address or the one where you intend to move to discover if you live close to one of the one thousand of the worst air-pollution zones.

2. **Do I live near a stationary plant releasing toxic chemicals into the air or water?** Put "Where You Live Environmental Protection Agency (EPA)" into a search engine, and use the nationwide map identifying nearby releases of chemicals that are part of the Toxics Release Inventory.

3. **Do I live near a nuclear plant?** Some fifty-five nuclear plants with ninety-three reactors are operating in twenty-eight states.[8] Many more operate in Europe and Asia. Visit Carbonbrief.org, and use their global map to track nuclear plants throughout the United States and the world.

I've gone to the Nuclear Regulatory Commission to obtain a list of active US plants.[9] Is there one in your neighborhood?

## US Active Power Reactor Units

| Plant Name | Location | Owner/Operator |
|---|---|---|
| Arkansas Nuclear 1, 2 | 6 miles WNW of Russellville, AR | Entergy Nuclear Operations, Inc. |
| Beaver Valley 1, 2 | 17 miles W of McCandless, PA | Energy Harbor Nuclear Corp. |
| Braidwood 1, 2 | 20 miles SSW of Joliet, IL | Exelon Generation Co., LLC |
| Browns Ferry 1, 2, 3 | 32 miles W of Huntsville, AL | Tennessee Valley Authority |
| Brunswick 1, 2 | 30 miles S of Wilmington, NC | Duke Energy Progress, LLC |
| Byron 1 | 17 miles SW of Rockford, IL | Exelon Generation Co., LLC |
| Callaway | 25 miles ENE of Jefferson City, MO | Ameren UE |
| Calvert Cliffs 1, 2 | 40 miles S of Annapolis, MD | Constellation Energy |
| Catawba 1 | 18 miles S of Charlotte, NC | Duke Energy Carolinas, LLC |
| Clinton | 23 miles SSE of Bloomington, IL | Exelon Generation Co., LLC |
| Columbia Generating Station | 20 miles NNE of Pasco, WA | Energy Northwest |
| Comanche Peak 1 | 40 miles SW of Fort Worth, TX | TEX Operations Company LLC |

*(Continued on next page)*

| Plant Name | Location | Owner/Operator |
|---|---|---|
| Cooper | 23 miles S of Nebraska City, NE | Nebraska Public Power District |
| D.C. Cook 1 | 13 miles S of Benton Harbor, MI | Indiana/Michigan Power Co. |
| Davis-Besse | 21 miles ESE of Toledo, OH | Energy Harbor Nuclear Corp. |
| Diablo Canyon 1 | 12 miles WSW of San Luis Obispo, CA | Pacific Gas & Electric Co. |
| Dresden 2 | 25 miles SW of Joliet, IL | Exelon Generation Co., LLC |
| Farley 1 | 18 miles E of Dothan, AL | Southern Nuclear Operating Co. |
| Fermi 2 | 25 miles NE of Toledo, OH | DTE Electric Company |
| FitzPatrick | 6 miles NE of Oswego, NY | Exelon FitzPatrick, LLC/Exelon Generation Company, LLC |
| Ginna | 20 miles NE of Rochester, NY | Constellation Energy |
| Grand Gulf 1 | 20 miles S of Vicksburg, MS | Entergy Nuclear Operations, Inc. |
| Hatch 1 | 20 miles S of Vidalia, GA | Southern Nuclear Operating Co., Inc. |
| Hope Creek 1 | 18 miles SE of Wilmington, DE | PSEG Nuclear, LLC |
| La Salle 1 | 11 miles SE of Ottawa, IL | Exelon Generation Co., LLC |
| Limerick 1 | 21 miles NW of Philadelphia, PA | Exelon Generation Co., LLC |
| McGuire 1 | 17 miles N of Charlotte, NC | Duke Energy Carolinas, LLC |
| Millstone 2 | 3.2 miles WSW of New London, CT | Dominion Generation |
| Monticello | 35 miles NW of Minneapolis, MN | Northern States Power Company – Minnesota |
| Nine Mile Point 1 | 6 miles NE of Oswego, NY | Constellation Energy |
| North Anna 1 | 40 miles NW of Richmond, VA | Dominion Generation |
| Oconee 1 | 30 miles W of Greenville, SC | Duke Energy Carolinas, LLC |
| Palo Verde 1 | 50 miles W of Phoenix, AZ | Arizona Public Service Co. |
| Peach Bottom 2 | 17.9 miles S of Lancaster, PA | Constellation Energy Generation, LLC |
| Perry 1 | 35 miles NE of Cleveland, OH | FirstEnergy Nuclear Operating Co. |
| Point Beach 1 | 13 miles NNW of Manitowoc, WI | NextEra Energy Point Beach, LLC |
| Prairie Island 1 | 28 miles SE of Minneapolis, MN | Northern States Power Company – Minnesota |
| Quad Cities 1 | 20 miles NE of Moline, IL | Exelon Generation Co., LLC |
| River Bend 1 | 24 miles NNW of Baton Rouge, LA | Entergy Nuclear Operations, Inc. |

| Plant Name | Location | Owner/Operator |
| --- | --- | --- |
| Robinson 2 | 26 miles NW of Florence, SC | Duke Energy Progress, LLC |
| Saint Lucie 1 | 10 miles SE of Ft. Pierce, FL | Florida Power & Light Co. |
| Salem 2 | 18 miles S of Wilmington, DE | PSEG Nuclear, LLC |
| Seabrook 1 | 13 miles S of Portsmouth, NH | NextEra Energy Seabrook, LLC |
| Sequoyah 1 | 16 miles NE of Chattanooga, TN | Tennessee Valley Authority |
| Shearon Harris 1 | 20 miles SW of Raleigh, NC | Duke Energy Progress, LLC |
| South Texas 1 | 90 miles SW of Houston, TX | STP Nuclear Operating Co. |
| Summer | 26 miles NW of Columbia, SC | South Carolina Electric & Gas Co. |
| Surry 1 | 17 miles NW of Newport News, VA | Dominion Generation |
| Susquehanna 2 | 70 miles NE of Harrisburg, PA | Susquehanna Nuclear, LLC |
| Turkey Point 3 | 20 miles S of Miami, FL | Florida Power & Light Co. |
| Vogtle 2 | 26 miles SE of Augusta, GA | Southern Nuclear Operating Co. |
| Waterford 3 | 25 miles W of New Orleans, LA | Entergy Nuclear Operations, Inc. |
| Watts Bar 1 | 60 miles SW of Knoxville, TN | Tennessee Valley Authority |
| Wolf Creek 1 | 3.5 miles NE of Burlington, KS | Wolf Creek Nuclear Operating Corp. |

4. **Am I downwind from a fossil-fuel power plant?** About 3,400 fossil-fuel power plants operate in the United States.[10] Type "Graphing Power Plants and Community Demographics" into an online search engine to get the link to the EPA's detailed map of fossil-fuel plants nearby where you live.

   (More than 2,400 coal-fired power plants operate in 79 countries.[11] Use the globalenergy.org world map to determine whether a coal-based power plant is in or near your community.)

5. **Do I have a coal ash plant in my community?** The United States has 738 coal ash plants in 43 states and Puerto Rico and thousands of unlined ponds whose heavy metal contaminants could well migrate into aquifers. Use the interactive "Mapping the Coal Ash Contamination" at Earthjustice.org to find out if there's a plant or pond near your home.

   Though not nearly as well publicized as other toxic issues, it's vital for you to know if you live near a coal ash contamination site.

The Environmental Integrity Project and Earthjustice have identified the most contaminated coal ash sites nationwide. You can find this report at https://environmentalintegrity.org/wp-content/uploads/2022/10/Poisonous-Coverup-11.03.22.pdf.

Here are the ten most contaminated sites (starting with the worst) that the report identified:[12]

**#1: San Miguel Plant** Christine, Texas
**#2: Reid Gardner Generating Station** Moapa, Nevada
**#3: Naughton Power Plant** Kemmerer, Wyoming
**#4: Jim Bridger Power Plant** Point of Rocks, Wyoming
**#5: Allen Steam Station** Belmont, North Carolina
**#6: New Castle Generating Station** New Castle, Pennsylvania
**#7: Brandywine Ash Management Facility** Brandywine, Maryland
**#8: R. D. Morrow, Sr. Generating Station** Purvis, Mississippi
**#9: Hunter Power Plant** Castle Dale, Utah
**#10: Allen Fossil Plant** Memphis, Tennessee

6. **Is there an ethylene oxide plant in my neighborhood?** Ethylene oxide is one of the most carcinogenic substances ever studied. Type "EPA Ethylene Oxide Information Page" into a search engine to visit their detailed listing of local facilities.

   In a survey released in 2022, the EPA announced locations of some twenty-three sterilizer facilities that pose a high local cancer risk. Being informed is the first step in self-protection. Do you live in one of these towns? If so, the self-protection methods, to be detailed shortly, will be vital to your family health. Here are the worst of the worst locations:
   Lakewood, Colorado
   Groveland, Florida
   Taunton, Massachusetts
   Hanover, Jessup, and Salisbury, Maryland
   Jackson, Missouri
   Columbus, Nebraska
   Franklin and Linden, New Jersey
   Ardmore, Oklahoma

Erie and Zelienpole, Pennsylvania

Añasco, Fajardo, Salinas, and Villalba, Puerto Rico

New Tazewell and Memphis, Tennessee

Athens and Laredo, Texas

Sandy, Utah

Richmond, Virginia.

7. **Are there oil and gas wells near our home?** The EPA, which supposedly protects our environment, approved forever chemicals' use in the oil and fracking industries because they repel water and make chemical mixtures stable and efficient. In the United States, about 1.7 million oil and gas wells (including those utilizing fracking-extraction methods) were active as of 2017, and about 12 million people lived within half a mile of these sites.[13, 14] Fracktracker.com provides an online interactive map to help pinpoint oil and gas sites in your community.

8. **Are you nearby railroad tracks?** The oil and chemical industries are sending tankers filled with explosive, toxic crude oil, vinyl chloride, pesticides, and other poisons via rail by the homes of more than twenty-five million Americans. Find out if your community is at risk by visiting the website Stand.earth/resources/do-you-live-in-an-oil-train-blast-zone and entering your address into their highly detailed map.

9. **Is the local water supply safe?** Go online to the local water supplier. Most provide testing reports of various usefulness and quality. Keep in mind utilities don't routinely test for PFAS, phthalates, or other unregulated chemical toxins. Prescription medications, solvents, pesticides, and antibiotics that make their way into drinking water systems are not subject to testing.[15]

The interactive map from the National Drinking Water Alliance at https://www.drinkingwateralliance.org/new-map tracks media reports of contamination. Pick your geographic locale and read the local news reports.

If you're on a budget and not planning on moving, I strongly urge you to save your money and spend it on water filtration rather than testing. (I'll share how to effectively filter your home's tap water in chapter 11.)

However, if you're moving and trying to find out about the local water quality, you can test the water of a prospective home. Mytapscore.com offers a pick-and-choose testing menu with guidance for both city and rural water supplies. Since PFAS taint as many as one in three taps, it makes sense to do a relatively inexpensive test for these chemicals. Cyclopure.com offers PFAS testing for under eighty dollars. The test kit, purchased online, comes with collection tubes and self-mailer.

Any amount of solvent, industrial chemical, pesticide, disinfectant byproduct, PFAS, heavy metal, or nitrate is reason to not live there.

10. **Do you live on or near a military or other Pentagon installation?** Two-thirds—some 266 of 389 Department of Defense sites in the United States where PFAS have been detected in groundwater—are contaminated with levels above federal health guidelines.[16] If you live near a military or Pentagon installation, it's likely your tap water is tainted. Visit the Environmental Working Group website and navigate to their interactive map detailing PFAS-impacted communities.[17]

11. **Is there a cell-phone tower in your neighborhood?** Knowing this is especially important before you move into a new community. However, no government regulations require carriers to publicize their 4G or 5G tower locations. The Federal Communications Commission, which regulates cell carriers, only requires them to register towers taller than two hundred feet. Most cell sites don't reach that height and are attached to light poles or placed on top of buildings.

To find out where cell phone towers are located in your local community, you should know about Network Cell Info Lite (for Android), which uses crowdsourced 4G and 5G data from Mozilla Location Services. Once you open the app, go to the map tab. You'll see nearby towers with a blue line to the one you're using.

Once you have gathered all of this information, you can take steps to protect your family.

## Close the Windows

Close your windows. If you live in the shadow of an industrial plant, that may mean keeping them closed. Otherwise, keep them shut during high-exposure periods. Do you live along or near a busy road? Shut your windows when traffic is dense. If your home or apartment is near a dry cleaner, for instance, close the windows when the wind blows toxic fumes into your domicile. One study of outdoor pollution's impact on air quality in homes during wildfire season found

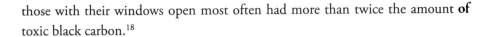

those with their windows open most often had more than twice the amount of toxic black carbon.[18]

## Filter Your Indoor Air

Outdoor pollutants become highly concentrated once trapped inside your home. An air filter is an essential survival tool in polluted communities. Studies show a mother's exposure to urban air pollutants during pregnancy damages a child's IQ. These chemicals are released into the air from the burning of coal, diesel, oil, gas, and tobacco. Cars, fracking sites, and factories are contributors to a child's IQ loss.[19]

In a study of pregnant women living in highly polluted environments in Ulaanbaatar, Mongolia, high-efficiency particulate air (HEPA) filters were used from around the eleventh week until the end of pregnancy in one group and none in the other. The IQ of children who were assigned to the air-filter group was almost three points higher.[20]

A HEPA filter can be purchased online for as low as thirty dollars. Be sure the filter you purchase is adequate for the size of the room for which it's intended.

When used properly, HEPA filters reduce particulate pollution by 99 percent as well as the overall risk of viral transmission.[21]

## Not Just Another Potted Plant

Potted indoor plants like golden pothos and ficus also help purify indoor air. House plants remove benzene, trichloroethylene, formaldehyde, and other airborne chemical toxins. The top ones for removal of chemical toxins are palms (areca, dwarf date, lady), bamboo; *Ficus elastica* and *Ficus maclellandii*; *Dracaena*, English ivy, Boston fern, and peace lily.[22, 23]

## Plant Trees

Growing trees around your home or on your balcony in large pots is another way to filter bad air. Silver birch, yew, and elder capture air particles via the hairs of their leaves and reduce pollution up to 79 percent.[24, 25, 26]

## Take Shoes Off Outside

Only about a third of us take off our shoes when entering the house.[27] Most of us would never insist our guests do the same before coming inside our home. But maybe we should. Using a doormat to stamp off your shoes reduces pesticides and other pollutants.[28] But even better is taking your shoes off entirely.[29]

## *Have a Home Emergency Kit*

Many families have emergency preparedness kits in case of natural disasters. But these kits should be augmented in the event there is an industrial accident in your area. In case of a train derailment or other kind of toxic event at a chemical plant, for instance, you should have full face mask respirators for each family member. Full face mask respirators filter out the smallest volatile organic chemicals present in polluted air. They cost from thirty to one hundred dollars and can be purchased online in adult and child sizes as well as for pets. Potassium iodide tablets are also a smart provision in the event of a nuclear accident since they inhibit the body's absorption of radioactive contaminants.[30]

## *Consider Protective Supplements*

Discuss the use of protective supplements for both you and your kids with a qualified health professional. I mentioned having an emergency supply of potassium iodide to block the body's absorption of radioactive particles in case of a nuclear accident. But taking potassium iodide regularly, as advised by a health professional, may be essential if you live nearby or downwind from a nuclear plant.

A published, peer-reviewed study shows the cholesterol-lowering medical drug cholestyramine, taken with chlorella, a single-celled healthy algae sold as a dietary supplement, reduces the body burden of PFAS.[31]

If one has high PFAS, the drug must be obtained through a doctor's prescription and chlorella from a health food store.

Chlorella supplements are also known to help the body excrete dioxin, a highly toxic industrial chemical.[32]

Antioxidants from the phytochemicals present in plants, along with vitamin and mineral supplements, help protect children from pollution. These can include herbs (turmeric, grapeseed, and green tea extracts), mushrooms and seeds like maitake and flax, and seaweeds such as brown kelp.

Susan and David Wind are members of a fast-growing family of parents who know the pain of having a chemically assaulted child and deeply inadequate, if not hostile, public support.

She wanted to know throughout the early days of her ordeal where the EPA was on all of this. Why wasn't the EPA protecting Taylor?

As time passed during the pandemic, Susan enlarged her vision.

"I wanted to create a movement of activist moms and dads to reform a broken system," Susan said on one of our phone calls.

"God knows, this country needs to reckon with its millions of chemical-assault victims. I'm going to do everything I can to protect our kids."

Susan spent hundreds of hours on the phone and email to connect activist moms across the country. She worked with the group Scientists, Activists, and Families for Cancer-Free Environments (SAFE) to bring moms together to make their voices heard.

Activist moms (and dads) from all over the country gathered at Freedom Park, in Arlington, Virginia, on September 20, 2022, for the nation's first-ever WE'RE HERE TOO demonstration on behalf of the millions of chemically assaulted families across our land.

Susan spent weeks making the signs—with life-sized lettering that read, "EPA: Do Your Job"—that the demonstrators carried when they marched across the Potomac River, interrupting traffic, to the agency's headquarters in Washington, DC.

They called on EPA to start enforcing environmental laws. They met with their congressional representatives and officials from the EPA and Centers for Disease Control and Prevention and called for better laws that actually work for the people to protect their children and punish polluters.

"The point is we're starting to feel our power," Susan said. "And we're communicating with each other to grow our movement. We're angry. We're so tired of inaction. But we're going to win because the people are with us. These issues transcend politics. Coal ash doesn't care if your kid is the daughter or son of a Republican or Democrat."

One of the moms who attended the September 20, 2022, WE'RE HERE TOO event and met with Susan and representatives at the EPA was the 2021 Goldman Environmental Prize winner Sharon C. Lavigne, another mother trying to keep her own six kids, twelve grandchildren, and community safe. Sharon didn't speak at the event, but her presence there completed the circle and brought together all regions of the nation.

Sharon, whose activism didn't begin until she was in her sixties, grew up in St. James Parish, Louisiana, along the Mississippi River, in an area known by the rest of the nation as Cancer Alley, some 85 miles with more than 150 industrial factories and chemical plants that stretch from Baton Rouge to New Orleans.

Today, when she drives through the parish, instead of the pastures of cows and beans of her childhood, she sees chemical storage tanks and smoke clouds.

Sharon began teaching special education students in 1982. Although there were always students who needed help, over nearly four decades of teaching in the local schools, she began noticing the number increasing.

I spoke with Sharon about the signs and symptoms she saw and associated with the toxic chemicals infiltrating her community's air, water, and soil. She began recalling students and describing them for me.

"I had one student in high school whom I recall—she was from Vacherie with pretty, long soft dark hair, who was slow with low scores in reading and math that could never pass those of a fifth-grade student," Sharon said in her soft southern drawl. "Another boy from Vacherie seemed to be pretending he didn't know a lot. That was because his mother wanted that disability check. But, as it turned out, he wasn't pretending. I remember three boys, all slow in math and reading. I have had kids with autism and just a lot of kids who were slow. I knew they were being hurt by the chemicals, kind of giving into the pollution, not because they wanted to; they were marginal kids, and pollution harms the low-income, vulnerable children the most. Their bodies are the least nourished, brains the least stimulated. The damage is so much more. Here, in our parish, no one wanted to solve the problem or know much about what was happening because special education students were a source of funding. The chemical companies make up the tax base here that pays for their education, perpetuating an insidious, vicious cycle."

When another polluting plant—the proposed Formosa Plastic Corporation factory—was slated for development in St. James Parish—and would have destroyed historic graveyards—Sharon began writing letters to public officials and invited community members to meet and organize at her home.

At first, folks met in her den but moved to the garage when their numbers increased. She founded RISE St. James, a faith-based environmental justice group that would eventually partner with Earthjustice and the Tulane University Law Clinic to file litigation to stop the Formosa plastic factory from further decimating her embattled community.

The people of the parish are winning this fight.

In April 2022, the EPA opened its Office of Environmental Justice and External Civil Rights. The office immediately began a civil rights investigation into the treatment of the families of Cancer Alley and also the Louisiana Department of Environmental Quality over the air-quality permits that were approved for the Formosa factory in both St. James and adjacent St. John the Baptist parishes.

In September 2022, Judge Trudy White of Louisiana's 19th federal Judicial District in Baton Rouge canceled the state-issued air permits needed to continue the project.

"The blood, sweat and tears of their ancestors is tied to the land," wrote Judge White. "Their ancestors worked the land with the hope and dream of passing down productive agricultural untainted land along the Mississippi to their families."

Judge White further noted that state regulators used "selective" and "inconsistent" data and failed to consider the pollution effects on the predominantly African American community.[33] However, a state appellate court in Louisiana overturned Judge White's decision in January 2024, and the case now awaits further legal review.

Sharon knows communities of color continue to bear disproportionately higher rates of toxicity. There's so much more to do, which is why she's working with the youth of her community to help them carry on the fight against a racist system of politicians, laws, and regulators who continue the state's historic attacks.

"They want us dead here," she said. "They want us to die out. But we're not going anywhere. This is our home."

The fastest pathway and impetus for change is when the people speak and make their actions heard. We speak with our votes, demonstrations, letter writing, testimony, and every day with our shopping dollars.

Did you know we don't need oil for all things plastic?

I know. I visited Natureworks in Blair, Nebraska, some thousand miles from Cancer Alley.

I toured the plant. I saw plastics being made using methods of fermentation without any harsh catalysts, petrochemicals, or toxic waste. Most folks don't connect plastic with oil. Almost everything in our lives that's plastic comes from oil. It doesn't have to be that way. We can move the market.

The plant, a project of Cargill, the largest private agricultural company in the nation, and Dow Chemical, provides local jobs and adds value to the corn crop. Additional plants have been built in Thailand, the Netherlands, and Japan. Other corporations operate such plants in Brazil where sugarcane is used.[34, 35]

Perhaps, if there were to be another plant in the parish, a non-polluting one using sugarcane would provide more local dollars flowing into the community and make a smarter, more environmentally sound choice.

NatureWorks' brand is called Ingeo, and it's being used for cosmetic cases, cups, takeout containers, serving ware, clothing, and bedding. Search for Ingeo and other bioplastics when you shop. Less toxic everyday products are now being manufactured, which is so much healthier for our children and local communities like St. James Parish.

Plastic without petroleum.

Life without cancer.

Healthy kids everywhere.

Imagine.

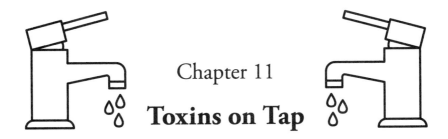

# Chapter 11
# Toxins on Tap

A sign, covered with ancient barbed wire, lost in time, proclaims, "Village of Hoosick Falls, Home of New York State's Best-Tasting Water 1987."[1]

It's a relic of a more innocent era in the life of a village that fell through the cracks of society's toxic safety net.

Starting in 1955, Hoosick Falls, nestled along Highway 22 near the New York–Vermont border, was home to eleven manufacturing plants providing more than five hundred good-paying, blue-collar jobs that were the "economic lifeblood" of the community. The men and women who worked at the plants produced fabrics, foils, yarn, and tapes. But what made these products unique was that they were stain- and water-resistant.

In the late 1990s and early 2000s, a flood of Middle Eastern petrodollars poured into the community to the tune of some $90 million in contracts to produce the flame- and water-resistant white tents for pilgrims who travel to Mina, Saudi Arabia, during the Hajj.

Work like that provided jobs for John ("Ersel," as friends and family called him) Hickey, who drove a school bus by day and, for thirty-two years, worked the night shift from 11 p.m. to 7 a.m at the Saint-Gobain Performance Plastics plant on McCaffrey Street. John's teenaged son, Michael, also worked at the plant during the summers. The plant sat on a hill. Nearby were the town's water wells.

The plants shared something in common: use of perfluorooctanoic acid (known interchangeably as PFOA or C8 for its backbone of eight carbon atoms attached to fluorine), synthesized in 1936, and one of the early members of a family of some six thousand or more molecular cousins known as per- and poly-fluorinated alkyl substances (PFAS).

Around town, the people complained about the foul-smelling tap water and riverbanks covered with orange goop. People were pretty sure the gooey mess came from the manufacturing plants. But everyone was making money.

John was in the first year of retirement in 2010 when his doctor diagnosed him with kidney cancer. Michael shared his story of visiting John the day his son Oliver was born in the same hospital where his father lay in bed with tubes all around him after losing a kidney to cancer.

"The moment was bittersweet to see life and death mingle so unnaturally," Michael recounted. "I raised a son who would hardly come to know his grandpa."

John "Pop" Hickey, surrounded by his loving family, drew his last breath in 2013. He will be missed every day by a son and grandson who were robbed of what should have been many more loving years together.

Heartbroken—worried over his family—Michael went on Google and researched "Teflon," discovering a report that would open his eyes to the data the DuPont company had long kept under wraps: a court-appointed panel overseeing the medical portion of the unfolding tragedy in Parkersburg, West Virginia. One of the chemicals identified coming from the factory was PFOA. The scientific tome of research confirmed kidney and testicular cancer were prevalent among exposed persons.

Michael went to the mayor, then county, and state officials to discuss getting the town's water tested. The mayor was concerned about reviving the town's economy, Michael told me. The plants that once made them well-to-do were on their way out one by one. Michael's news wouldn't be good for the economy, he was told.

Another public official reminded Michael no federal or state law required towns as small as Hoosick Falls to test their water.

Michael hired the same company testing the water in Parkersburg to analyze samples at his home, mother's residence, McDonald's, and Dollar Tree. The lab discovered high levels of PFOA in all of the tests including 540 parts per trillion (ppt) and 460 ppt at Michael's and his mother's homes, respectively. High levels were found at the commercial sites, too. There is no known safe level for chronic exposure to durable carcinogens like the PFAS family, and that is particularly true of PFOA, the most intensively studied of them. He shared his story in December 2015 with the *Times-Union*, which broke the news, shaking the town to its core.[2]

Hoosick Falls males are being struck by testicular cancer with the same alarming frequency found in Parkersburg, West Virginia. Michael reeled off three recent cases when we spoke.

"One involved twenty-eight rounds of chemotherapy. Another person I spoke to was forty-seven years old. His testicle was removed yesterday."

In an email to then New York Congressman Antonio Delgado (now the state's lieutenant governor) and activist groups, Michael wrote Hoosick Falls needed more help. He said he hoped to put together a more aggressive game plan for medical monitoring.

"We need screening and education for testicular cancer in the high schools of contaminated communities," Michael wrote. "We need to educate and prepare young people who may move out of a once-contaminated community for the possibilities of illness down the road. Forever-chemicals mean the possibility of getting sick is always there. A better understanding of future illnesses must be taught at a younger age to create earlier detection by self-examinations. My concern is if people move out of Hoosick Falls and their life evolves, they forget about the exposures they grew up with."

By attending the 2019 State of the Union address with Representative Delgado and testifying four times in Washington, Michael continued to shine light on his community's experience as a symbol for the many towns across our land now facing PFAS contamination.

Although no PFAS-specific bills made it out of the 2019 Congress, the National Defense Authorization Act (NDAA), which passed that summer, contained provisions requiring a phase-out of PFAS use in military firefighting foam and food packaging; all air and water discharges of PFOA were to be made public under authority of the Emergency Planning and Community Right-to-Know Act of 1986.

The NDAA also directed the Environmental Protection Agency (EPA) to decide whether to add other PFAS to the nation's Toxic Release Inventory within two years. Finally, the legislation required that, under the Safe Drinking Water Act, larger public water utilities would need to begin testing their water supplies.

Michael took the lead in civil litigation that helped compensate the community in 2022 with a $90 million–dollar settlement including a new clean water supply and bio-monitoring for citizens at a regional facility in Vermont.[3] Nearby Petersburgh and Bennington, Vermont, which faced similar contamination issues, were part of a larger umbrella settlement.

"I'm not your typical environmentalist," Michael admitted. "I'm not a natural born activist. I'm a quiet underwriter. I like my cubicle life." He laughed. "But the quiet person can be an activist, too. At least, that's what I have learned and one of the things I share with others in my situation. You don't have to be the stereotypical loud person to become an activist. When I am speaking to high school classes, I share with the kids there are more opportunities now for people like me who are quiet to make a difference. I tell them that you don't need to be the person carrying the sign. There are ways for the quiet guy in the back of the room who can have an impact by doing the research, following through, and believing in the cause. I hate public speaking. But I surrounded myself with the right people. I believe, by establishing the new water supply and bio-monitoring, we have a road map for the future."

But where is justice? The people of Hoosick Falls enjoyed an important court victory that demanded accountability; however, now they face a lifetime of anxiety over the specter of the possible long-term health effects from their toxic exposures. In a very real sense, no amount of money could possibly restore the families of the town to what they once had in that sweet time, back in 1987, when they were innocent, and Hoosick Falls could proclaim it had the best-tasting water in all of the state of New York.

## Toxins on Tap—A Family Protection Plan

There is no such thing as safe chronic exposure to any amount of lead, pesticides, phthalates, PFAS, industrial solvent, or chlorinated disinfectant that causes cancer or reproductive toxicity. Zero tolerance is the only way to protect your health.

### Filter Your Water

Every home in America should filter their tap water. Unfiltered tap water is especially dangerous during pregnancy and causes a higher rate of miscarriages and complications.[4]

For families on a budget—and what one today isn't?—I'd rather have them use their financial resources to purchase protection instead of testing.

Every home should have an under-the-sink (or countertop) reverse osmosis (RO)–based system that uses additional filtration methods to cover a wide range of contaminants.

Many models can be self-installed and retail for under three hundred dollars.

Duke University and North Carolina State University scientists say many systems they tested were only partially effective at removing PFAS. Those systems using carbon filtration alone were among the least effective. The RO models were extremely effective.[5, 6]

Key takeaways from their study include:

- Activated-carbon filters removed 73 percent of PFAS contaminants, on average, but results varied greatly. In some cases, the chemicals were completely removed; in others, they were not reduced at all. Changing out filters regularly is essential to their ability to reduce PFAS.
- The PFAS-removal efficiency of whole-house systems using activated carbon filters varied widely. In four of the six systems tested, some PFAS levels actually increased.
- However, under-the-sink RO with two-stage filters achieved near-complete PFAS removal. Reverse osmosis combined with two-stage filters reduced PFAS levels, including newer compounds like GenX, by 94 percent or more.

Here are the units the Duke University and North Carolina State researchers found have the highest proven reliability:

The free-standing, pre-plumbed, five-stage iSpring RO system comes with both booster pump and color-coded feed and discharge tubing. It was tested over a seven-day period. All PFAS in the effluent were reduced below detection for the entire test period. Plus, you can install their systems yourself.[7]

The four-stage Flexeon RO System was also pre-plumbed. All PFAS in the effluent were reduced below the detection limit for the entire test.[8]

Aquasana AQ-5200 (not in the study) is certified by the National Sanitation Foundation (NSF) to significantly reduce some seventy-seven different contaminants, including lead, mercury, volatile organic compounds (VOCs), and pharmaceuticals. The system is one of a handful of filters certified for PFAS removal. Filters need to be replaced every six months at a cost of one hundred twenty dollars per year. Being barely larger than a couple of cans of soda, the system doesn't take up a lot of valuable room under your sink.

If your budget is really strapped, a faucet-mounted system for under thirty dollars can reduce both heavy metals and PFAS. One faucet-mounted carbon filter made by PUR was tested for seven PFAS chemicals typically seen in groundwater in

Washington County, Minnesota.[9] The system reduced six of the seven below 5 to 10 ppt. The other was reduced by 75 percent.

In yet another study, NSF-approved, faucet-mount filters for heavy metals were tested in homes and businesses in Flint, Michigan.[10, 11] Without filtration, the lead concentration of the water was an average of almost 3 parts per billion (ppb) but, filtered, went down to less than 1 ppb.

Optimally, you want to use several different filtration methods. A combination of under-the-sink RO with faucet-mounted and pitcher filters is a good health plan.

Consider the following:

**Use a filter pitcher.** Brita, Pur, ZeroWater, and similar filter pitchers are affordable to a huge demographic and make an invaluable contribution to public health. Because of PFAS contamination, you might consider using the NSF-certified Purefast filter cartridge made from plant sources in your Brita pitcher. They cost forty-five dollars and filter up to sixty-five gallons. (Each Purefast cartridge comes with a package and prepaid label to return the filter to the company. The contaminants will be converted into salts and safely disposed without harming the environment.) On the other hand, the new ZeroWater pitcher removes PFAS too and retails for under thirty dollars. (This is what we're currently using in our fridge and the model the Healthy Living Foundation delivered to residents in St. James Parish as part of a program there to improve drinking-water quality.)

**Distillation is extra insurance.** At our home, we also use a WaterWise countertop distillation system. Distillation removes 99 percent of PFAS and most other contaminants.[12]

**Filter your shower, garden, and other faucets.** Showering and bathing leads to the absorption of PFAS, pesticides, and solvents. One study found inhalation and skin exposure to VOCs from showering was equivalent to ingesting around two liters or quarts of water.[13] Shower filters remove both VOCs and some PFAS. These sell for under thirty dollars too and take ten minutes to install. Replace your shower filters regularly.

Filters for garden hoses are available for around twenty-five dollars and should definitely be used if your water is contaminated with PFAS and other toxic compounds.

**Let tap water run for thirty seconds to two minutes.** The first flush of water from your faucet contains the most lead and any other accumulated contaminants.

Let the water run up to two minutes for the worst heavy metals and toxic chemicals to flow out.

Systems that can effectively remove PFAS are also likely to perform best for heavy metals, solvents, pesticides, industrial chemicals, and other contaminants. Please, have tough standards for your home drinking water. Same for the water your family uses for bathing and even gardening. An effective home water filtration system may seem expensive. It isn't. Not really. No matter where you live, a home drinking–water filter system is the best health insurance policy you will ever purchase.

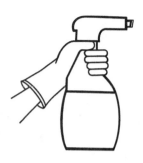

# Chapter 12

# Homesick

Seventeen-year-old Jessica Cabrera, of Salinas, California, loved her Sunday morning house-cleaning ritual with her mom, Martha.

"It's a fun time," she said. "We sing lyrical rhymes together, dance, and make complete fools of ourselves as if we were performing in front of a raging crowd at a dance fest."

But Jessica also worried her mom's loyalty to her old ways of cleaning were hurting their health.

"I see it. I smell it, and I feel it," she said. "There is a constant stigma of cleaning being an essential hygienical need, but we never hear about how to properly do it the healthy way."

Jessica's mom "suffers from a thyroid condition," she said.

Jessica was a teenager when she became one of the youth research assistants in the Lifting Up Communities with Interventions and Research (LUCIR) study in Salinas that examined how to reduce toxic exposures from cleaning products. (*Lucir*, in Spanish, means "to show or shine light.")

Now that Jessica knew so much more about cleaning products and the impact of the endocrine disrupting chemicals (EDCs) they contained on thyroid health, she worried their frequent use could be exacerbating her mom's condition.

One day, Jessica spoke to her mom about cleaning their home and its health impact. It was as if she was shining a bright Hollywood Klieg light on health issues Martha had never thought about before.

"I told her about all the repercussions I have noticed and have had an effect on her," Jessica said. "I knew we had to make a change in what we use, how we do it, and what we can do to take preventative measures."

The next morning, Martha, in a jacket and ready to go out, awakened her daughter with a croissant.

"Let's go to the store and help me pick out some products."

The LUCIR study is yet another partnership between the CHAMACOS Youth Council, La Clinica de Salud de Valle Salinas, and the researchers at the UC Berkeley School of Public Health.[1] This time, the Salinas teens decided to study the toxicity of cleaning products being used by members of their local community.

"One thing I learned is Latina women are more exposed than most persons to harmful chemicals from cleaning products," says Youth Council member Stephanie Mayo-Burgos, coauthor with Jessica of the peer-reviewed scientific paper they published with their CHAMACOS colleagues and UC Berkeley scientists in *Environmental Health Perspectives*.[2]

Stephanie, majoring in Environmental Studies and Legal Studies at UC Santa Cruz, cited three underlying statistical factors she and the other investigators uncovered during the course of the study that were causing higher toxic exposures among Latina women: social status, education, and culture.

"Some 81 percent of professional household cleaners in California are Latinas," she said. "That means at least 160,000 women are being exposed all day long five days a week in California alone. That's a lot of exposures with consequences, even more if you include their family members, and the many women who may actually be pregnant when they're cleaning. I also see what's happening in this state is occurring across the nation. We are the fastest growing population in the country, and we have to educate our people through any means possible. As a Latina, I can say we grow up with the scent of clean and the brands our mothers used. Conventional cleaning products are heavily scented to fool us into thinking clean has to have a scent."

The LUCIR study has helped Stephanie's own health. "I have had allergies since I was a kid, so the products my mom would buy were making them worse. I didn't know the cleaning products with all their fragrances were causing my breathing difficulties. Then I became involved with the LUCIR study and learned about the toxic effects of cleaning products."

Jessica, Stephanie, and the other teens recruited women from the shopping centers, medical offices, nearby hospital, and other meeting spots in Salinas. The women they recruited were largely Latina. The teens offered prospective participants free nontoxic products and a fifty-dollar gift card if only they would wear a small, lightweight backpack for a period of time while cleaning. The backpacks had air monitors and measured chemicals being emitted by their cleaning products. The teens prepared each air-monitoring pack.

The backpack air monitors measured the women's exposures while they cleaned their homes using toxic products for one week and then again with the "green" brands.

The air samples were analyzed for forty-seven chemical toxins of concern because they were EDCs or on California's Proposition 65 list of carcinogens and reproductive and developmental toxins.[3]

The study proved interventions work and have a lasting impact on our cleaning habits, which, in turn, helps raise healthy kids. Switching to safer products led to significant decreases in exposure to seventeen chemicals of concern including some particularly bad ones like 1,4-dioxane, chloroform, benzene, naphthalene, toluene, and hexane. The women who participated in the study said the replacement products worked equally well.

"We conducted a survey six months later and learned nearly two thirds of the women had begun using almost totally all-green products, and 95 percent were using some with their cleaning," Jessica said.

A few chemicals like terpenes and musk went up, though. But this is because even some of the green products used perfumes, fragrances, or other scents. Switching to non-fragranced products could have eliminated these exposures.

Because kids spend so much time at home—some children as much as 90 percent of their day and night—the quality of their indoor air matters. If it becomes filled with dust and airborne chemicals from cleaners, cosmetics, furnishings, bedding, clothing, dry cleaning, insecticides, air fresheners, electronics, and more—that, truly, is enough to make a child homesick.

## Homesick—A Family Protection Plan

The first step in cleaning up your home is easy. Get rid of the bad actors. I've examined the major brands such as Ajax, Lysol, Mr. Clean, Soft Scrub, Clorox, Planet, Simple Green, Fabuloso, and Windex—they all use glycol ethers, quats, ethoxylated alcohols, dyes, and fragrances. None are safe for use during pregnancy or by persons of reproductive age, or, really, by anybody else who cleans regularly or for extended periods.[4, 5, 6, 7] You should throw these products out if you're pregnant or want to have children. And, if you're pregnant, have someone else slip on protective gloves and respirator and take them to a hazardous-waste collection site.

There's good news, though. Safe brands are similarly priced and clean equally well.

The testing the Healthy Living Foundation (HLF) has performed for toxic chemicals of concern shows one brand in particular, ECOS, has earned much-deserved praise for producing safe and healthy formulas.

At *Healthy Living* magazine, a HLF publication, we commissioned a lab to test two different products—ECOS Parsley Plus All-Purpose Cleaner from Earth Friendly Products and Simple Green's All-Purpose Cleaner—in an airtight chamber for emissions of toxic volatile organic chemicals (VOCs). One would think a product like Simple Green should be fairly healthy, right? After all, you would think it's "simple green" branding implies environmental sensitivity. Simple Green emitted ten times more VOCs (many of them toxic) than ECOS Parsley Plus, which cleaned just as well, if not better. In yet another study HLF performed of some two dozen laundry detergents, ECOS tested free from any detectable amounts of the dangerous chemical 1,4-dioxane, which causes breast and other cancers.

I visited the ECOS manufacturing plant in California. The company has four of them, strategically located in Washington state, Illinois, New Jersey, and California, to reduce transportation-related greenhouse emissions. Once inside their solar-powered plant, the air quality was excellent. There were no smells of solvents or other chemical toxins being stored anywhere on the premises. The workers, I learned, are paid well and have benefit packages. The company was the creation of the late Van Vlahakis, among the most important and notable green chemists in our time. Van came to America as a penniless teenager, a World War II refugee from Greece. As a student living in Chicago, Van waited on tables while acquiring a degree in chemistry from Roosevelt University. Instead of later working for manufacturing companies "dumping" formaldehyde and toxic solvents into cleaning products, which he knew was a highly dangerous and reckless practice, he used his knowledge to create Earth Friendly Products and the ECOS brand that has grown into one of the most popular lines in the nation.

Sadly, I lost my friend Van in April 2014. He loved the sea, boats, and the fresh ocean breeze. Nothing brought him more joy than boating with his granddaughter and sharing his love for the blue waters of his homeland.

Fortunately, for all families, Van's dream and vision live on. Kelly Vlahakis-Hanks, the company's vice president, succeeded her father as president and chief executive officer. Kelly continues the company's commitment to safe cleaning products, sustainability, and zero waste. She has become widely acknowledged for her leadership in the green movement and corporate social responsibility. Under her guidance, ECOS may well be the world's first company to produce its goods in carbon-neutral, water-neutral, and zero-waste-certified facilities.

Other brands to favor include Dr. Bronner's and Better Life. I use both of these companies' products, too. These brands truly are safer, better, and less toxic.

The same chemicals in cleaning products strictly regulated in "workplaces" face little if any scrutiny when used in our homes. Although the Cleaning Product Labeling Act of 2017 requires disclosure of ingredients on the label, many websites make it impossible to know what's in the product before purchasing. Amazon.com is one of the worst websites for information about the ingredients in its cleaning products. Sellers' websites frequently lack this information, making it difficult, if not impossible, for shoppers to know what's inside the product they're purchasing.

We're all busy with ever-lengthening to-do lists. No one has the time to do all of the research—looking up ingredients and investigating which of them are toxic—necessary for family protection.

That's why I've done the work for you and gone ahead and rated the most popular cleaning brands. All you need to do is arm yourself with this information and reach to your left instead of the right for the safe choice.

# Safe and Unsafe Home Cleaning and Laundry Brands

🛒 = Safe, none, or least risk from chemical toxins

⬤ = Dangerous, contains significant amounts of chemical toxins

| Product Name | Reproductive and Developmental Toxicity | Cancer |
|---|---|---|
| Ajax | Dangerous | Dangerous |
| All | Dangerous | Dangerous |
| Arm & Hammer | Dangerous | Dangerous |
| Better Life | Safe | Safe |
| Boulder | Dangerous | Dangerous |
| Cheer | Dangerous | Dangerous |
| Clorox | Dangerous | Dangerous |
| Comet | Dangerous | Dangerous |
| Dr. Bronner's | Safe | Safe |
| Dreft powder | Safe | Safe |
| Easy Off | Dangerous | Dangerous |
| ECOS | Safe | Safe |
| Era | Dangerous | Dangerous |
| Gain | Dangerous | Dangerous |
| Green Works | Safe | Safe |
| Ivory | Dangerous | Dangerous |
| Kaboom | Dangerous | Dangerous |
| Life Tree | Safe | Safe |
| Lysol | Dangerous | Dangerous |

*(Continued on next page)*

| Product Name | Reproductive and Developmental Toxicity | Cancer |
|---|---|---|
| Method | | |
| Microban | | |
| Mop & Glo | | |
| Mr. Clean | | |
| Mrs. Meyer's | | |
| Oxiclean | | |
| Planet Ultra | | |
| Pledge | | |
| Puracy | | |
| Purex | | |
| Seventh Generation | | |
| Simple Green | | |
| Sun Burst | | |
| Tide | | |
| Tide Free | | |
| Tilex | | |
| Weiman | | |
| Wisk 2x Ultra | | |
| Woolite | | |
| Woolite Complete | | |
| Zep | | |

## *Quick and Easy Homemade Formulas*

You can make a few simple homemade formulas to cover most situations.

Try these quick and easily prepared homemade cleaners instead of Lysol, Windex, Formula 409, and Fantastik! They're less expensive, work better, and don't expose your kids or baby to stealth chemical toxins.

**Simple All-Purpose Cleaner (instead of Formula 409):** Combine ½ cup of distilled white vinegar with 2 cups of water in a spray bottle.

**Germ Slayer All-Purpose Cleaner (instead of Lysol):** Mix 2 cups of water, ½ cup of white vinegar, 2 tablespoons of rubbing alcohol with 6 drops of peppermint, rosemary, or lavender essential oil in a spray bottle.

**Tough Job Surface Cleaner (to replace Fabuloso and Mr. Clean):** Mix 2 cups hot water, ½ cup distilled white vinegar, 1 teaspoon of washing soda, and 1 cup Dr. Bronner's liquid soap in a spray bottle for a formula that cleans as well as the purple stuff.

**Hello Sunshine Glass Cleaner (to replace Windex):** Mix 2 cups of water with a ¼ cup of white vinegar and ½ teaspoon of Dr. Bronner's liquid soap to get cleaner windows than with the blue-dyed bomb.

**Non-Harsh Oven Stain Cleaner (to replace Easy Off):** Sprinkle baking soda, moisten with water. Let stand overnight. Wipe and clean.

**Fabric Softener (instead of Febreze and Snuggle):** Replace quat-loaded fabric softener dry sheets by adding 1 cup of distilled white vinegar to the rinse cycle to prevent static cling, soften, brighten, and reduce odors.

Can we talk about dust, the great Trojan horse of your home? Dust contains all of the traces of chemicals from everything we bring into our dwelling. It's literally a forensic history of your home. The cosmetics, cleaning products, electronics, furniture, bedding, toys, soles of your shoes, work clothing, and just about anything else you bring into your home will sprinkle their most durable and toxic chemicals into your dust.

Dust accumulates the poisons in your home. When you live in a dusty home, you inhale more poisons. This might seem trivial. It isn't. Dust is a significant contributor to toxic exposures for babies, infants, and children.[8]

To pass the white-glove dust test is easy once you have a game plan. Here's yours for a healthy, low-toxin home:

**Use a high-efficiency particulate air (HEPA) filter and vacuum.** I discussed in chapter 10 how important a HEPA filter is to a healthy home. A HEPA room filter reduces the amount of airborne nanoparticles and VOCs circulating indoors. However, floors, especially carpeting, harbor potential mini-dust storms of toxicity we inhale into our lungs. Using a HEPA-based vacuum is the most effective method of removing fine particles embedded in carpeting and beats steam cleaning for removal of pollutants and allergens including lead and pesticides.[9, 10] Vacuuming without a filter removes lead but not as much (if you can't afford the more expensive HEPA models).[11]

**Replace furniture with flame retardants.** Seek furnishings and textiles with either Oeko-Tex or European Naturtextil IVN certifications that limit petrochemicals, including per- and polyfluoroalkyl substances (PFAS), and require the use of organic or other natural and sustainable materials.[12]

Furniture manufactured earlier than 2020 could contain undisclosed flame retardants. Send a small foam sample for a no-cost analysis to the Duke University Foam Project at https://foam.pratt.duke.edu/. If the test is positive for their presence and you want to keep your furniture, replace the cushions with safer flame-retardant-free materials.

In 2020, California banned sales of upholstered furniture, juvenile products, and mattresses containing most flame retardants and required they have labels to inform shoppers of their presence.[13] Many companies sell their California furniture nationwide. The information tag is usually located beneath the cushions or on the bottom.

Ashley Furniture, Endicott Home, Ethan Allen, and Crate and Barrel furnishings are free from flame retardants.

**Replace toxic home and garden pesticides.** Do not store or handle Ortho, Raid, Black Flag, Roundup, and other similarly toxic products if you're pregnant or have children. Have someone else take them to a hazardous-waste collection site. Wear nonpermeable gloves and full face respirator when handling.

If you use a gardener or lawn-care company, be sure to talk with them about what they're using. Make sure they aren't using pesticides and herbicides like Roundup (glyphosate), 2,4-D, carbaryl, or any of the pyrethroids in their sprays and fertilizers. If they do, that's dangerous. Trugreen.com and Naturalawn.com offer nationwide organic and natural methods for pest and weed control.

## Safe and Unsafe Home and Garden Pesticide Brands

🛒 = Safe, none, or least risk from chemical toxins
🛒(dark) = Dangerous, significant amounts of chemical toxins*

| Product Name | Reproductive and Developmental Toxicity | Cancer |
| --- | --- | --- |
| All-Purpose Home Insect Control | Safe | Safe |
| BioAdvanced | Dangerous | Dangerous |
| Black Flag | Dangerous | Dangerous |
| Bonide All Seasons Horticultural & Dormant Spray | Safe | Safe |
| Clean Green | Safe | Safe |
| Earth's Ally | Safe | Safe |
| EcoLogic | Safe | Safe |
| Ecovenger | Safe | Safe |
| Green Gobbler | Safe | Safe |
| GrowSafe | Safe | Safe |
| Mosquito 3-in-1 Killer | Safe | Safe |
| Natria | Safe | Safe |
| Ortho | Dangerous | Dangerous |
| Roundup | Dangerous | Dangerous |
| Safer | Safe | Safe |
| Scotts | Dangerous | Dangerous |

**Toss Teflon pans.** It's probably time to toss any of those last remaining Teflon-coated fry pans and other cookware. On the other hand, traditional cast-iron and carbon-steel pans are safe. I like cast-iron because it's so versatile and lasts for generations. Like cast-iron, carbon-steel pans are versatile and can be moved from stovetop to oven and back again.

**Think glass.** Plastic chips and flakes. Those little nanoparticles become part of the dust stream. Least-toxic container materials include glass (think Pyrex), stainless steel, and lead-free ceramics.

**Don't sleep with the enemy.** Sheets, toppers, coatings, and your mattress can all be coated with PFAS besides other toxic chemicals. Seek bedding without stain- and water-resistant claims. Organic latex, cotton, down, and wool are all available for bedding and mattresses. Wool is also highly flame resistant.

Avocado, Awaraa, Lifekind, Saatva, Parachute, Birch, Coyuchi, Plush Beds, Brentwood Home, Bear, and Spindle offer organic and sustainable materials in their bedding.

**Go perc free.** Carbon dioxide ($CO_2$) molecules that make soft drinks fizzy can also be used to safely clean clothing. The process, known as wet cleaning, uses $CO_2$-infused water. It outperforms other alternatives including perchloro-ethylene, the solvent used in dry cleaning, which is toxic to the fetus, and gives clothes that peculiar ether-like smell when you bring them home.[14] Get wet with your new cleaner at Nodryclean.com.[15]

**Goodwill hunting.** Vintage clothing manufactured before the 1970s is likely to be PFAS-free and safer and certainly better for the environment than toxic fast fashion with petrochemicals, dyes, and waste.[16] Used clothing has been washed so many times, the toxic finishes have been eventually laundered out. Find vintage fashion brands at great prices at Goodwillfinds.com, the online outlet for the nonprofit Goodwill Industries

**Prefer slow fashion.** While fast fashion relies on highly toxic processes and chemicals such as dyes, alcohol ethoxylates, and PFAS—"slow fashion" is a far more sustainable and less toxic choice.

Organic clothing and fashion are available from Poetry.com, Harvestandmill.com, Peopleheartplanet.com, and Pact.com. Jockey offers organic undergarments and exercise clothing. (Jockey organic lounge and workout sweatpants are the bomb!) Cariuma and Rothy's shoes are eliminating toxic chemicals from their footwear.

Organic and sustainably sourced children's clothing includes Honest Baby, Carter's, Hanna Andersson, Touched by Nature, and Pact.

Seventh Generation, Kudos, Coterie, NatyBaby, and HealthyBaby are all striving to create the least toxic diaper.

**Leave work clothing at the job.** If you work at a job where toxic materials are used, your employer should be offering industrial laundering for safety purposes since chemicals in trousers and other clothing are prime ways to bring chemical toxins into the home and expose your children to them. If your employer doesn't launder work clothing, leave your items outside your home, and wash separately.

**Buy toxic-free toys and other household items.** Check before you buy toys and other household products to make sure they're free from polyvinyl chloride (PVC), the chemical toxin released in the tragic East Palestine, Ohio, train derailment. Rubber chickens, bath ducks, wading pools, beach balls, bibs, backpacks, and anything soft, plastic, and pliable will harbor PVC.[17] Toys or products with recycling code #3 contain the poison.

Black plastic toys, more than any other color, contain the highest concentrations of heavy metals that are comparable to coal ash from waste incinerators. This is because black plastic, used in making electronics, has long been impregnated with toxic flame retardants.[18, 19]

Choose organically sourced cotton stuffed animals and unpainted wooden blocks and toys. Seek toys made from solid wood, organic textiles, and other natural materials. Make sure your baby's pacifier is made from natural rubber and free from bisphenol-A (as in "BPA-Free") and all of the other BPA-related compounds.

The next time you shop for new household items such as a shower curtain, for example, avoid those stating they're made with PVC. Instead, choose a product made with polyethylene vinyl acetate (PEVA). Although not perfect by any means, PEVA is certainly a safer material that is free from highly toxic chlorine molecules.[20] Better yet, if your budget allows, buy an organic cotton shower curtain, woven for thickness and density to repel water and dry fast.

Most garden hoses are made from PVC. Kids and pets drink from such hoses. But they shouldn't.

There are safer garden-hose alternatives. Look for ones like the lead-safe, high-flow Big Guy; Armadillo; and GatorHyde. These hoses are made from polyurethane, which, again, isn't perfect—but, at least, PVC-free. Choose hoses made from recycled polyurethane whenever possible.

The green cleaning revolution the CHAMACOS youth began in Salinas during the pandemic "is so much larger," Stephanie said excitedly during one of our conversations. "We created a series of animated videos, voiced them ourselves, and did many media interviews during the pandemic, including an in-depth story with the Union of Concerned Scientists, to share our findings nationally. But the most important method of change, we found, came from word of mouth.

"The women in our study told their friends about using nontoxic cleaning products. That was huge. When one of our study participants went green, she told others; they told their families, and the message spread. The women from our study are educating their friends and children, the scent of clean may be no scent at all. Some products are so heavily scented, they fool us into thinking that's what clean smells like when really the facts show how bad these products are for our health. I'm not saying things are perfect here by any means, but I also see changes leading to improvements in community life. We're disrupting the culture in our town in a good way. I feel empowered to be one of the persons making that change."

We vote every day with our shopping dollars and can use them to fuel environmental justice for all communities.

I try not to be too tough on myself. You shouldn't be too tough on yourself either. But do we really need to risk a PVC release like the one that occurred after the February 4, 2023, train derailment in East Palestine, Ohio, just for a garden hose or plastic ducky?

I know I can do better. We can just resolve to shop smarter now that we know more—whether we're buying cotton shower curtains or PVC-free baby bibs!

We can buy tablecloths made from safer materials than those plastic PVC-soaked, stain- and water-resistant ones. The same goes for our kids' backpacks that we buy every fall when they return to school. We don't have to opt for petrochemical-heavy cleaning products, either. We can become even more aware—(dare I say, more "woke"?)—and push the market and society in a safer direction to give all families improved lives.

Together, when all of us make smarter choices about what we bring into our homes, that's one way we can cast a powerful vote to end the toxic madness.

# The World Beyond
# Our Front Door

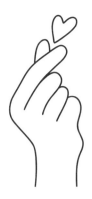
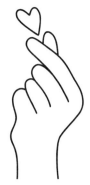

# Chapter 13

# New School Rules

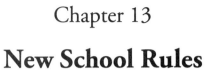

Andrea and Joe Amico were full of hope and anticipation when they decided to move from Massachusetts to the Seacoast region of New Hampshire in 2007. The couple wanted to be closer to Joe's work where he was employed as a visual designer for a business located at the Pease Tradeport in Portsmouth.

Twenty miles of sandy beaches and rocky headlands, from Salisbury, Massachusetts, in the south, to the Piscataqua River and Kittery, up north in Maine, made for stunning sights driving the last stretch to their new hometown.

Four years later in 2011, Andrea and Joe were blessed with their first child. After months on the waiting list, they were thrilled to learn of an opening at Great Bay Kids Co., one of the two daycare centers next door to Andrea's husband's workplace. Joe could drop off their daughter and pick her up.

"It was a beautiful facility with brightly colored classrooms and loving teachers," Andrea recalled. "Joe could see the window of our daughter's classroom from his office and would stop by on his lunch break to feed her a bottle or take her for a walk."

Their second child, a son, was born in 2013. Like his older sister, he started daycare when he was twelve weeks old.

In May 2014, on a Friday before Memorial Day, the *Portsmouth Herald* newspaper reported high levels of per- and polyfluoroalkyl substances (PFAS), used for firefighting at military installations, had been found in the Haven Well that supplied drinking water to her husband's office and kids' daycare at the Pease Tradeport.[1]

"I thought of my husband and two small children who were on Pease for work and daycare every day and drinking the water," Andrea said and paused, reliving a primal feeling of personal guilt.

Andrea remained quiet and listened, seated alone in the very back row at the first community meeting that local and state public officials hosted to discuss the issue of PFAS in the town's well. One after the other, so-called experts told everybody the presence of PFAS in their children's water posed minimal risk. Andrea felt compelled to ask questions and wanted to know if there would be blood testing to see who had been exposed. No, they weren't going to test anybody, she was told. No, it was too expensive. Not needed. It's not routine.

But nothing was routine anymore, and it was not all right.

Andrea was certain of two things: That first meeting would not and could not be the last. And she would no longer sit in the back of the room and take it.

But there was also a lot to learn.

"Pease was one of the first communities in the nation to learn its members had been exposed to high levels of PFAS as a result of the military's longstanding use of aqueous film-forming firefighting foam," Andrea told me with a voice fueled with anger, pain, and resolution. "I was totally out there dealing with the unknown. Most of all, we needed to know what to do to monitor our health and be proactive in diagnosing and treating adverse health effects that might result from our PFAS exposure, and no one would help us with that."

Andrea began engaging with the health department about testing and where she could get answers for her concerns over the possible long-term effects of PFAS on her children and husband.[2] But after seven months of trying to get answers, Andrea and her family felt the sting of a nonresponsive, uncaring, and unhelpful public agency.

Things changed, though, when Andrea contacted New Hampshire Senator Jeanne Shaheen in Washington, DC, who became actively involved and made the necessary calls to get the testing done. Then, in early 2015, Andrea shared her story in the *Portsmouth Herald*.[3, 4]

"The article led to a chain reaction and jumpstarted the movement that finally led to PFAS blood testing for the community," Andrea said.

Andrea and her family spent a few fun days at Lake Winnipesaukee, the most expansive inland body of water in the state, in July 2015. When they got home, they were tired but happy. Joe was lugging in their bags filled with wet towels, and the dogs were barking.

Andrea spotted four large, yellow envelopes mixed in with the rest of the mail on the kitchen counter. A lump stuck in her throat, and a pit formed in her stomach. She opened each with dread.

Joe and the children had high levels of PFAS in their blood. Their daughter, Sophia, then almost five (now twelve), had the highest.

"I will never stop worrying about the health of my children, and I will forever live with the guilt I unknowingly sent them to a daycare center where they drank contaminated water," Andrea told me remorsefully. "When I stop to think about just how contaminated the water was my family drank and compare it to the updated Environmental Protection Agency (EPA) advisories, it is daunting and heartbreaking my young children were exposed to that much poison and they will live with these chemicals in their body and may experience subsequent health effects from what they drank as babies and toddlers at daycare. It's incredibly unfair to all of the Pease community members who were contaminated without consent—poisoned without permission. My family members are guinea pigs in an experiment we did not sign up for. It makes me mad and feel guilty all at the same time. But it's what fuels me to keep fighting, too. There's so much work to be done."

Andrea cofounded the community action group Testing for Pease with two other mothers, Alayna Davis and Michelle Dalton. Their work quickly evolved into advocating for the entire Pease community to better understand the long-term health impacts from PFAS exposure. Their advocacy led to the nation's first federally funded PFAS study to monitor the health effects on the Pease families.

Contaminated drinking water is just one of the stealth issues confronting schoolchildren today. Most kids don't have much choice when it comes to which school they attend. Yet, they spend some seven hours a day there. That's more than one thousand hours a year.[5] More time is accrued if kids participate in before- or after-school programs.

It's common sense we shouldn't build schools on or near toxic waste sites and factories, especially since we know how damaging pollution is to academic performance.[6, 7, 8, 9, 10] But we do so all of the time. [11, 12, 13, 14]

We shouldn't be spraying herbicides and pesticides on campuses either, given all of the neurological damage they do to school-age children. But pesticides are widely used including on the grounds of our colleges and universities.[15, 16]

Reducing each student's toxic exposures, as well as teaching them about self-protection methods, should be part of the new core curriculum for every school.

## New School Rules—A Family Protection Plan

Is your school in a danger zone? Obviously, no one wants their children to attend schools by busy roads or bus stops, smokestacks, oil wells, military installations, waste dumps, Superfund sites, and other nearby sources of harmful emissions.

Put "EPA Toxics Tracker" into your search engine. Enter your school address into the database to learn of nearby industrial facilities with toxic emissions.

However, many hazardous waste sources are abandoned properties and no longer reporting their emissions. To find out if your school was built on a toxic, abandoned industrial property (often known as a "brownfield") or near a Superfund or other hazardous site, enter the address into the EPA database "Cleanups in My Community."

Here's what you need to do if your school is located by sources of dangerous toxic emissions:

**Shut your classroom windows.** For schools located nearby acute air pollution sources such as rush-hour traffic, it is advisable to keep windows and doors closed during peak pollution periods. (If outdoor pollution levels are low, open windows or doors to help ventilate the classroom.)

**Use an air filter in the classroom.** Just as I discussed the importance of healthy indoor air for your home in chapters 10 and 12, school classrooms should also be free from pollutants. If your school is located by smokestack industries and other pollution emitters, it may be necessary to keep the windows closed most, if not all, of the time. An open window provides the best ventilation. Otherwise, use a high-efficiency particulate air (HEPA)-based filter. Many school districts began providing classrooms with HEPA systems due to the pandemic.[17, 18] But, if not, and the school won't provide them, as outrageous as that may be, parents might need to pool their resources to purchase a system for their children's classroom or classrooms. These filters might be larger than one purchased for home, since a classroom may be larger in size.

**Place indoor plants in the classroom.** Indoor plants are another smart idea for reducing classroom pollution. Start with easy-to-grow ones like jade, English ivy, and golden pothos. Palms and ficus remove toxic chemicals too.

**Check the school's water quality.** Tainted school tap water is a pervasive health problem. It isn't just PFAS, either.

The Federal Government Accountability Office reported in 2018 less than half (43 percent) of schools had tested their drinking water. Of schools that reported results, 37 percent found unacceptable levels of lead.

Stel Bailey, a concerned mom and director of the nonprofit organization Fight for Zero that monitors for PFAS and other sources of contamination in Florida, did an independent survey, submitting public record requests to sixty-seven school districts and forty-two colleges to request drinking water test results.

"We learned some counties hadn't tested their drinking water in decades," Stel said.

A school may offer you a report from the local water supplier. But this isn't adequate. Lead contamination often occurs after water leaves treatment plants and mixes with antiquated pipes. Your school should have reports of the water quality coming out of its own taps.

But what if your school has no tests? You should demand the school do its own testing, and if they won't that might not be a good school to stay at. As with home water testing, a simple flask is all you need to test what's coming out of your school's taps and water fountains. It's unfair, but perhaps the classroom or PTA parents can pool their resources if their school is indifferent to children's health and test or filter the classroom water. Any kind of lead, solvents, pesticides, or PFAS is reason for concern.

Kids should avoid drinking water and beverages and eating foods made at school or nearby places. I'd even be concerned over kids showering there or joining the water polo or swimming teams if the water has any kinds of contaminants. Kids can always do a dry shower, if required by school rules or hygiene. I'd even be concerned over recreational pools in the area.

**Give your child safe water to drink from a stainless steel flask in cases where school water is contaminated.** Keep it simple. Be careful when shopping for insulated flasks. Lead-based solder is used with most of them to seal in the vacuum layer. Hydroflask, an insulated water bottle, is lead-free.[19]

**Protect your kids if they ride a bus to school.** Most of the nearly half-million school buses, which carry more than twenty-three million children, use diesel fuel. How can kids excel when they inhale the vapors of diesel fumes as if they were sniffing glue or vaping? Diesel exhaust causes cancer, IQ loss, and poor academic performance.[20]

The situation can be worse for kids with asthma or chemical sensitivity. If your child must ride the bus, here are ways to lessen their toxic burden:

- Windows should stay open whenever weather permits.
- Avoid sitting in the rear over the exhaust.
- Sit in front, the place of least exposure.

**Don't add to your child's toxic burden.** Be sure children's preschool and kindergarten nap mats are made without flame retardants. The nonprofit group Toxic-Free Future found when childcare providers replaced nap mats with chemical-free versions, levels of flame retardants in kids' bodies decreased by 90 percent.[21] Today's mats are largely free from flame retardants. Those made before 2014 could well have them. Mats sold in California must bear a label stating whether they have flame retardants.[22] Since products sold in California are often offered nationwide, the mat you're using or about to purchase may well have such a label. It's worthwhile looking for ones that do to be assured no flame retardants were used.

## Have You Seen the Lights?

The illnesses at Sky Valley Education Center, in Monroe, Washington, were too prevalent to ignore. They seemed to have begun in 2014.

Besides headaches, arm and leg rashes, skin cysts, and oral blisters, the students, staff, and parents who visited the school suffered mental declines and uterine cancer. A six-year-old little girl experienced puberty. The health effects were terrifying.

School officials, apparently, were vacationing in the state of denial, displaying supreme negligence in caring for students and staff.

Teachers used fans to clear the air inside classrooms when the school's fluorescent lights began to emit fumes. They used buckets to catch oil dripping from their ballasts onto desks and floors. The only thing left to do was to evacuate the school and test that darkened gunk.[23, 24]

It was loaded with polychlorinated biphenyls (PCBs). Although banned since the 1970s because they cause cancer and damage the fetus, PCBs are still found in capacitors used for cooling in school lighting ballasts. The school's light ballasts, needed to regulate electrical current to the decades-old fluorescent lights in the classrooms, were filled with one of the most child-toxic chemicals known to humankind and leaking like sieves.

Unfortunately, despite district claims in July 2021 that its PCB mess had been cleaned up months before, by January 2022, the *Seattle Times* and *ProPublica* reported an EPA spokesperson claimed the agency was still waiting for a cleanup plan before it could make a "formal decision." Fines, further cleanup, or approval of the yet-to-be-submitted plan were options. The kids are back at school, anyway, some, no doubt, looking up at the lights every now and then.

Twenty-eight percent of all currently active public schools were built before 1950, 62 percent between 1950 and 1984, and 10 percent after 1985.[25] Schools constructed before 1980 are likely to have PCB- and asbestos-containing materials.

For these reasons alone, it pays for you to be alert to your school's maintenance and repair activities. These durable synthetic toxins and materials may be lurking behind wallboards, ceiling tiles, or caulk dust in about half of all schools.

The good news is PCBs and asbestos are usually contained unless maintenance, repair, or construction activities occur. The bad news is many thousands of kids currently are being exposed to either or both.

Be alert to construction or maintenance occurring in auditoriums, classrooms, corridors, restrooms, and teachers' lounges. Removing old caulking can lead to airborne PCBs. Leaking fluorescent light ballasts or simply ones that look old are another warning signal for possible exposure to PCBs.

Asbestos is also of concern, especially for schools constructed before the 1980s. Asbestos causes a cancer called mesothelioma, a cancer of the tissues surrounding the lungs. Maintenance we might think of as typical, like replacing ceiling tiles or opening a popcorn vault with trowled-on materials, should be of concern, especially if your school was constructed prior to 1980. The activity of even replacing older pipes and hot water tanks can cause asbestos fibers to become loosened, air borne, and distributed via the heating ventilation and air-conditioning system.

Take advantage of the Asbestos Hazard Emergency Response Act (AHERA) to find out if your school has an asbestos problem. Established in 1986 under the

Toxic Substance Control Act, AHERA requires all public, private, religious, and nonprofit schools to perform inspections in their buildings for asbestos-containing materials. Schools with asbestos issues must prepare a management compliance plan. You should know what your school's inspection report and any management plans say. Use this sample letter as a model to personalize your own request for this information.

> Dear Principal—,
> I am writing to obtain digital copies of the school's inspections of buildings for asbestos-containing materials and management plan. My request is made under authority of the Asbestos Hazard Emergency Response Act (AHERA).
> AHERA requires all school districts, including public, private, nonprofit, and religious, to adhere to certain guidelines to mitigate asbestos exposure risk. This includes inspections and a compliance-management plan should any asbestos be discovered. Thank you for your cooperation.
> Sincerely,

If your school has an asbestos issue, it's vital to instruct your children to stay away from cordoned-off areas undergoing maintenance or construction.

You also have other parental rights I want you to know about. Most of us have long believed if our child is attending a school campus with toxic threats they can't transfer to another school.

Yet, many educational districts allow student transfers during what is known as "open enrollment" period. These transfers can be requested for reasons from academic distress to health concerns (for example, an asthmatic child shouldn't go to a school that is located near smokestack factories) or being closer to where a parent works.

The National School Choice Week website, Schoolchoiceweek.com, offers insights into each state's rules for open enrollment.[26]

But it may be that you or your kids don't want to go to a different school, or open enrollment might not work out.

There's still a lot you can do to make sure your child is safe from toxic chemicals.

## *Start a Green Team*
Consider banding together with other like-minded parents to form a green team

for your classroom or school. Each parent can take on an individual task instead of everything falling on one person.

A green team is vital to a healthy school. You will get to know other parents, teachers, staff, and students. The bonds you form change the total nature of your school experience: the team process involves everybody, and you end up building strong, lasting ties.

The friendships I formed working with other parents at Topanga Elementary School, in our little mountain community, have become part of a support network that has lasted for years. I liked working on school projects with the parents who cared about the environment such as recycling, gardening, and trail, creek, and beach cleanups.

A green team can review cleaning and classroom supplies, food quality, use of pesticides, make sure the tap water is safe, and even schedule a trash pickup day to raise awareness among students.

The team can also help pressure school officials on other important toxic issues like use of landscaping pesticides, herbicides on sports fields, the health consequences of converting grass to synthetic turf, providing classrooms HEPA filters, or dealing with potential asbestos and PCB issues.

Invariably, expertise will be needed. Someone might be best at interpreting an asbestos report. Someone else could review what pesticides are being used and their toxicity. Yet another person might be in charge of making sure the equipment on the school playground is safe. It's great to know how capable other parents are and that you can count on each other to join together on behalf of the kids.

We all know how important a healthy, nutritious diet is to our children's physical and mental health. I've looked at school menus from Pacific Palisades, California, all the way to Montgomery, Alabama. The one thing they have in common is way too many foods, such as chicken nuggets and salads, with a high content of organophosphate (OP) pesticides, the brain and nerve toxins we learned about in chapter 1. If schools would only serve organically sourced fruits, veggies, and grains, kids' IQs, across the board, would go up.

But schools are notorious for serving pesticide-filled dishes with lots of enriched grains, chicken nuggets, burgers in fluffy buns, buttery muffins, beef tacos, and anemic salads with iceberg lettuce.

A green team can help put healthier foods into children's bodies. The Farm-to-School lunch program, headed by The Center for Food and Justice, can connect your school with local farms. They work with almost eleven thousand schools in more than thirty states. The schools that take part in this program buy farm-fresh, local foods, such as fruits, vegetables, eggs, and beans, and serve them in the cafeteria. To implement the program at your school, you can order a free information resource packet from the Farm-to-School website at Farmtoschool.org.

The green team can also help implement use of safe cleaning products. Responsiblepurchasing.org lists least-toxic products and where they can be purchased for professional janitorial uses.

Twenty percent of kids in the United States and Canada wear uniforms to school.[27] If their uniforms are stain-resistant, they're most likely absorbing PFAS through their skin. The frequency and duration of time kids wear their uniforms certainly raises concerns. (The same goes for outfits for the Girl Scouts and Boy Scouts as well as sports gear and other uniforms for extracurricular activities.) A green team can help source safer uniforms without claims they are stain- or water-resistant and positive assurances they're PFAS-free.

## *Leaves of PFAs*

Back in the early 2000s, when both moms had kids in preschool, Jean Bryant, a Seattle mother of three boys, was talking to her friend, Amy Griffin, who had two young sons of her own. Amy mentioned those "little black dots" that appeared on the synthetic turf their kids played on and seemed to be replacing natural grass throughout the country.[28] The little black dots were recycled tire crumbs sprinkled over synthetic turf to affect a natural feeling.

Amy, an assistant head coach of women's soccer at the University of Washington and the national and US Olympic teams, mentioned "it was weird" that many of her current and former players, especially goalkeepers, had been diagnosed with cancer.

"You don't think it has anything to do with those little black dots, do you?" she said.

Jean hadn't the faintest idea and didn't give Amy's comment a second thought.

But about a decade later, in 2015, on Mother's Day, a nurse called Jean after she had sent her son Jack, then fourteen, to the doctor because of a chronic cough.

The doctor found swollen lymph nodes in Jack's chest, and the nurse called to inform Jean her son had been diagnosed with Hodgkin's lymphoma.

Jean's job was to tell her beloved son he had cancer. "My commitment was not to break down in tears or to fall apart," she told CNN. "That wasn't my job as his parent. My job was to let him know it was going to be okay."

Jack continued to play soccer after his first cancer treatment in an effort to continue normal activities. But he relapsed, and he hasn't played on a soccer field since. But there's also good news. On June 20, 2020, Jack, then nineteen, having taken up other sports like basketball and baseball, received news that his "scans came back all clear, best gift ever."[29]

"No one at this point can convince me playing on ground-up tires is a healthy option for kids," Jean told the news organizations.

The majority of sports fields in the United States are switching to synthetic turf with crumb rubber contaminated by heavy metals and undisclosed PFAS (used to make the turf more durable). The little pepper flakes are mixed in with the turf to cover the field and simulate real soil. They are made from recycled tires and filled with cadmium, benzene, nickel, chromium, and arsenic. For kids who play on these surfaces, synthetic turf can become a significant source of toxic exposures.

The Washington State Department of Health offers tips on how to minimize potential exposures to chemicals from synthetic turf fields. These are the rules for your kids to follow whether they're playing on synthetic turf or playground equipment made with wood posts (usually preserved with arsenic or other pesticides that cause cancer):[30, 31, 32, 33]

- Always wash hands after playing on the field or other play structures and certainly before eating.
- Take off shoes to prevent tracking crumb rubber into the house.
- Be sure to shower after playing on the field and quickly treat any cuts or scrapes.
- Never swallow crumb rubber.

## That Talk

Have you had that talk yet with your kids? I mean the one about their smartphones.

Devra Davis, PhD, president of the Environmental Health Trust, a nonprofit group based in Jackson, Wyoming, has authored Disconnect, which explores the risks of 5G and cell phones. In her book, Dr. Davis has sounded the warnings on cell phone radiation and offers these safe-use guidelines that apply to our children as well as ourselves:

- Make sure your kids use anti-radiation headphones and are texting instead of taking calls. Anti-radiation headphones are designed to minimize electromagnetic field radiation; texting involves much less exposure, too.
- Kids shouldn't put the phone up against the side of their skull or in their pockets—except when on airplane mode.
- If they don't have headphones, they should use the speaker as far away from their body as possible.
- Tell your kids if they place their phone on their lap, use a barrier like a book or pillow to increase the distance between their body and the device and reduce exposure.
- All of us should keep cell and wireless phones away from babies, infants, toddlers, and other kids and adults.
- Children should never sleep with their phones. (Check to make sure the phone is nowhere near your child's head when they go to sleep at night.) They should turn it off or put it into airplane mode.
- Don't let your child carry their phone in their pocket or against their body when it's turned on. Males who use cell phones the most have the least sperm and worse quality compared to those with less radiation exposure.[34] Instead, kids should turn off their phones or place in airplane mode and keep them in their backpack or locker.
- Keep the back of the phone, where the antenna is located, facing away from the body.
- Kids should use their phone when and where the signal is good. In marginal areas, their phone requires greater power output so they are exposed to more radiation.

Finally, pregnant women should keep cell and wireless phones away from their abdomen. Mothers who use mobile phones the most during pregnancy are likely to have shorter gestation periods and more miscarriages.[35, 36, 37, 38, 39]

Kids like healthy school environments. Their brains and bodies aren't fooled when they know no one cares and their school environment is toxic.

The Inflation Reduction Act President Joseph R. Biden signed into law in 2022 has several important provisions for school environmental safety including providing funding for "protecting our children with investments to monitor and reduce pollution at public schools in disadvantaged communities."[40]

This law, together with the Infrastructure Investment and Jobs Act and American Rescue Plan, passed in 2021, will help fund the transition from diesel to electric buses; upgrade the pipes that deliver tap water to our kids while at school; replace boilers, ovens, and other appliances with clean-running models; and install solar and geothermal energy sources.[41]

Nonetheless, grant funding, from which K-12 schools benefit, represents less than 1 percent of overall spending in the most recent bill.[42]

That's why it's vital that you share what you've learned with other parents. Your voice and knowledge are needed.

We need everybody to be aware of what's going on in our kids' schools whether for bullying, troubled students, potential gun violence, or toxic hazards. We need everyone's eyes and ears.

There's so much to do in so many areas.

That's why it's so important for everyone to know the new school rules.

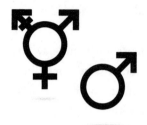

# Chapter 14

# Joy of Gender

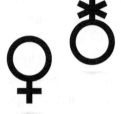

Growing up in the 1990s in St. Louis, Missouri, Mere Abrams had no concept of male or female. Mere's parents called them a tomboy. They pointed out the masculine influence of Mere's two brothers on their sibling. But Mere also had an older sister.

"I gravitated toward my brothers," Mere recalled. "It was all right, too. People liked tomboys. Tomboys were okay."

It was even okay with Mere's conservative Jewish parents when they joined the boys' basketball team and became their starting point guard. But not even that was enough to fit in.

"The boys did not respect that I was the starting point guard," Mere said. "Even though I earned my spot on the team based on skill, I noticed the boys did not want to pass me the ball. Even though I dressed like them, my lengthy, curly red hair (which my parents forced me to keep long enough to stay in a ponytail), was a clear sign I was not one of them (and they assumed that meant I would not be as athletic)."

Mere's parents never outright told their child to give it time, follow the rules of society, and everything would get straightened out when they were older. "But this was a message I picked up on based on being told that I had to wear a dress, bra, and other feminine clothing, fashion, and accessory items. I surrendered to the overwhelming feeling of eventually needing to 'be a girl/woman' and all the expectations that came with that notion."

Dad was a Missouri Republican at that time, mom a registered, blue-dog, pro-choice Democrat. They loved their kids, of course. That wasn't blue or red.

Mere turned twelve and began preparing for the Jewish coming-of-age ritual called a bat mitzvah (for girls) that involves memorizing portions of the Torah and performing them before a full congregation that usually includes not only close friends but every relative one has ever known, however distant.

Mere's mother took them shopping in downtown St. Louis.

"I want to wear a tuxedo," Mere said, leading their mom over to the men's section.

"No, dear. You have to wear a dress."

"But I can wear a boy's basketball uniform, so why not a tux?" Mere said.

"This is what you are required to wear when you're in temple," their mom said.

"Sure," Mere said, trying to be the child their parents wanted them to be.

"She reinforced the social expectation," Mere remembered.

Mere wore a satin sparkly dress at the bat mitzvah in front of what seemed like all of St. Louis's Jewish society when secretly they knew a tuxedo would have felt more natural. But Mere went through the whole ceremony presenting themselves as the girl everybody expected.

"I understood what society wanted," Mere added sadly.

That's how it went. Presentation became the *modus operandi* of Mere's teen life.

At that tender age, Mere kept hearing conflicting inner voices. One voice told the young teen the tomboy must go away. *Act like a female!!! You're a girl!!! Look at yourself in the mirror.*

*You must because you want to please Mommy and Daddy and live up to their expectations.*

"I really believed if I did everything my mom and dad wanted me to do, all of my dreams would come true," Mere recollected. "Based on the positive attention I received when I wore tighter clothes, I felt as if I needed to keep doing this."

St. Louis was dystopian. When Mere attended seventh grade in the early 2000s, Black kids were still being bused to white schools in an effort to integrate, and a diversity forum was held to talk not only about race but sexuality, particularly homosexuality, a word that seemed sinful and screamed out evil to the then seventh grader.

"To many people, talking about race felt threatening and uncomfortable. Sexuality stood out to me as something that was also a particularly hot button for certain people and families.

"You wouldn't believe how many of the parents wouldn't allow their kids to attend not because of race but due to the homosexuality portion of the program," Mere went on. "That was when I knew I was different. I began feeling different too. The word *homosexuality* kept sticking in my brain. It seemed so wrong. Yet, it was a door I had to open.

"But the word was so limited. It meant one thing. It didn't describe me," Mere said. "What made things difficult was lacking the words to articulate what was going on inside me."

"I had no queer friends," Mere recalled. "One boy I knew was femme but afraid to come out. Gender or sexual orientation weren't discussed at school or even between friends. It just wasn't done back then. If you did, you could expect to get mocked or harassed. So you just didn't talk about it with anyone."

Instead, Mere kept wearing dresses, dating boys, and trying to please St. Louis society.

"I felt like I was on an assignment I had to pass with flying colors. I wanted to conform because I wasn't aware of the life I could have been living," Mere said and seemed so lost.

Everything became internalized like a room without windows or any other escape paths. Mere's anxiety manifested in debilitating stomachaches that rendered the child prone and sick for hours in their bedroom. Mere recalled to me that the "anxiety became overwhelming."

There were points when boys flirted with Mere, but they weren't attracted to in return. Other times there were girl crushes. It was all very confusing. Mere kept thinking maybe it was just a phase that could be endured to reach some better place up ahead.

*Maybe I'm gay? Lesbian? Trans?* Mere wasn't sure. Mere had no one to talk to about the confusion and discomfort within their own skin. Mere wasn't depressed and suicidal like some kids became when they realized they were queer or identified as trans. Instead, Mere engaged in chest binding, a practice of flattening their breasts, which helped them feel better about themselves.

"It was still really difficult to talk about what I was going through and share my feelings with my family and friends," Mere told journalist Naomi Darom in *Haaretz*, an Israeli newspaper.[1] "I had all these preconceived notions of what it was like to be LGBTQ. I thought if you were lesbian, gay, or trans you would never have a partner or family. You would probably get kicked out of your house and become the target of bullying and harassment."

Mere told me: "I heard trans-identifying kids often ended up doing sex work or adult entertainment, none of which interested me. I also knew some kids became suicidal or hurt themselves. I had no thoughts of suicide or doing any harm to myself. It wasn't like I hated parts of me either. The traits and things I associated with being trans didn't seem like they would bring me any happiness. Only hardship . . ."

Mere turned eighteen and did what any suppressed, bright, questioning young adult living in St. Louis and identifying as lesbian, gay, bisexual, transgender, queer, or another sexual or gender variation (LGBTQ+) would do in the early 2000s: they left.

Mere went to California to study at The Claremont Colleges outside of Los Angeles. There, anyone could put on a skirt, walk on campus, and attend classes without raising an eyebrow. Every shade of the gender spectrum inhabited campus life.

"It was so liberating," Mere said breathlessly, remembering those times.

Mere began dating a girl, returned home to Missouri, and told Mom about the possibility they were "bisexual." Mom said she was okay with a "lesbian daughter" and hugged her child.

But that was strange. "I didn't tell my mom I was lesbian," Mere said. "I wasn't quite certain *lesbian* fit."

Dad, next, consulted the Old Testament. He reviewed the relevant passages and, when finished, said he had some very good news, indeed, for his beloved child.

"He noted Leviticus 18:22 and 20:13 only mentioned men when having relations with their own sex as being an abomination that 'they shall surely be put to death,'" Mere said wryly.

"Thank God it wasn't one of your brothers, right?" I replied.

"This was something I thought to myself but did not say out loud," Mere explained. "In that moment I didn't say much. I was just grateful I wasn't a disappointment to them.

"I'm not sure any of us understood it at all," Mere said. "It was still largely a mystery. I remember thinking that night, 'Okay, now my parents think I'm a lesbian, but that just explained attraction; it still didn't identify one's gender.'"

At one point, Mere joined a group of college girlfriends, all of whom were heterosexual, and flew with them to the Dalmatian coast of Croatia. It should have been a time for parties and moonlight dancing with days spent sunning themselves on the sandy beaches along the clear blue waters of the Adriatic. Instead, Mere became even more isolated and depressed.

"I left and flew home because, in the time I was there, it became clearer and clearer to me that I did not feel like one of them and did not want to have to continue pretending I did.

"I had to go and try one last time to be hetero," Mere said. "Instead, going on that trip and what happened, leaving everyone as I did, proved I was totally unable to be what people wanted or expected. I remember coming back home, now in my early twenties, and doing several entire days of meditation and self-reflection. After that, I went to a Ross department store and bought myself a pair of men's briefs. I always felt better in them even when I was a kid and would steal my brothers' briefs just to feel them against my skin. I went up to the cash register, feeling like the whole world was watching, and paid for them. I walked out and stepped into a new world."

Mere returned to California to start an internship that was part of the clinical social work program at San Francisco State University and began working on a graduate degree.

Finally, after so much searching, the word came: *nonbinary*. Mere finally knew they didn't have to be this or that gender. They could flow from feeling one way to another.

"Each step of my journey I know now, difficult as it has been, affirmed an important part of who I am," Mere said. "All I knew for certain was I didn't solely identify with the sex I was assigned at birth. There was more to gender than that."

Now a licensed clinical social worker practicing in Palm Springs, California, Mere told me emphatically, "I want kids to know it's okay to be scared. But kids also need to know they're loved and supported by their parents. Anyone with gender questions has a right to be able to get good counsel and factual information based on science."

Meanwhile, Mere's father, the former Republican, has become an active Democrat and, in response to hateful anti-transgender rhetoric, they shared with me, "He's one of the greatest allies of the LGBTQ+ community, speaking out against anti-trans legislation to everyone he knows whether they agree or not."

With all of the fashion issues Mere faced growing up, they bring a unique perspective to a new generation with Urbody, a line of stylish base layers, beautifully and sensitively designed for the needs of all variations of how persons gender identify and how their bodies are shaped.

"The reception to our site has been overwhelming," said Mere. "We're filling a growing need. A number of major fashion brands have consulted with me because of what we're doing at Urbody. They see how the fashion market is being shaped. They want to learn about how these changes in society intersect with fashion.

"Oh, there's more," Mere said excitedly. "I have a child with my partner, you know? And we're expecting a second baby in the next few months."

I never thought my passionate interest in environmentalism would ever lead me to conduct an in-depth investigation of how we gender identify and its enormous implications for raising healthy children. However, clearly, with the great amount of hateful legislation directed at the LGTBQ+ community, we absolutely must, as caring parents and citizens, understand the scientific basis for gender identification.

I first became interested in the influence of our environment on gender identity from an unlikely source: the alligators of Lake Apopka, the fourth largest freshwater body of water in Florida, and the scientific research of the wildlife reproductive biologist Dr. Louis Guillette.

After graduating with a doctoral degree in reproductive endocrinology in 1985, Dr. Guillette arrived at the University of Florida, whose mascot was Albert the gator, ready to get on with his new job, never knowing it would last a lifetime.

In those years, the state was trying to figure out whether alligator ranching could become a sustainable industry. Florida's longtime, legendary alligator expert, Allan Woodward, asked Dr. Guillette to take on the task of learning everything he could about the feasibility of such an endeavor.

Among the many sites Dr. Guillette visited, Lake Apopka's population was vastly different, with only a few juveniles and mainly adults who didn't seem particularly interested in reproducing. In nests at most lakes, he learned that 70 to 80 percent of the eggs were hatching. But when he reached Lake Apopka, some 80 to 95 percent failed. When gators emerged from those few eggs that did hatch, Dr. Guillette observed the penises of the male juveniles were only one quarter the normal size; mature males had testes that were flat and resembled ovaries. In some cases, the gators were born intersexed with both testes and ovaries. Typically, in healthy females, each follicle houses a single perfectly formed egg, but there were three or four prematurely released smaller-than-normal ones in the follicles of the Lake Apopka alligators. Levels of testosterone in infant and juvenile males were so out of proportion he figured they were probably sterile. In other cases, levels of testosterone were normal, but their hormone effect was being blocked.

Playing detective, Dr. Guillette couldn't help but observe on the shores of Lake Apopka the Tower Chemical Co. facilities with their abandoned buildings and rusting drums behind a series of chain-linked fences posted with signs that warned ominously "CONTAMINATED SITE."

Tower Chemical manufactured the pesticide dicofol for years with several major spills into the waters of Lake Apopka. Like my beloved Santa Monica Bay with our own DDT catastrophe, Lake Apopka would later be designated a federal Superfund site. Dicofol, unfortunately, is contaminated with up to 20 percent DDT, which is highly estrogenic.[2, 3]

Despite the intimidating appearance of the male gators, their reproductive systems were in a state of gender chaos. Over time, Dr. Guillette was able to show this effect was no doubt from the dicofol and DDT turning the lake's waters into a sea of estrogen in which the gators swam.

All vertebrates, that is, species with backbones, from alligators to humans, start out life with the potential to become either male or female, depending on their chromosomes. When we first begin as fetuses, our bodies simultaneously develop two separate kinds of tissues, one that gives rise to male and the other to female reproductive systems.

Early in the prenatal period, under the influence of a burst of sex hormones, a switch is thrown, and the proper set of tissues is signaled to develop while existing tissues fated for the opposite sex are designated to self-destruct. This is the job of the messenger chemicals that are part of the endocrine systems of all vertebrates. One such messenger chemical, Müllerian-inhibiting substance, is normally released in developing male vertebrates to cause the resorption of the embryonic tissues that would produce a female reproductive system.

However, small amounts of hormone-like chemicals from the environment, we now know, can mix with the sex hormones to perturb this precise hormonal ebb and flow, whether we are talking about Lake Apopka alligators, Missouri River sturgeon, Wisconsin frogs, California gulls, or our own children. In the lake's alligators, the chemicals were interfering with sexual development and causing varied intensities of feminization, defeminization, masculinization, and demas-culinization of males, females, and their few offspring. Lake Apopka's alligators had morphed into a third gender when compared to those untouched by toxic chemicals.

Our children's reproductive systems are as plastic as those of the gators. They change in relation to the environment too. They always have. It's just now with fake hormones so widely in circulation that it's happening in a novel manner—and to an entire population.

In 2009, neurobiologist Dick Swaab, former director of the Netherlands Institute for Brain Research, along with colleague Dr. Alicia Garcia-Falgueras, published an article in the peer-reviewed journal *Functional Neurology* that put forward as fact what only a few years earlier had been labeled a "premature" hypothesis: prenatal exposure to sex hormones affects brain development and gender identity—how persons identify themselves may even conflict with their genitalia.[4]

The doctors explained how the fetal brain develops in the male direction through the direct action of testosterone on the developing nerve cells or in the female direction through its absence.

"In this way, our gender identity (the conviction of belonging to the male or female gender) . . . [is] programmed into our brain structures when we are still in the womb," the doctors wrote.

They also noted that sexual differentiation of the genitals takes place in the first two months of pregnancy. The testosterone-influenced sexual differentiation of the brain, however, won't begin until the second half. This means "these two processes can be influenced independently, which may result in transsexuality. This also means that in the event of ambiguous sex at birth, the degree of masculinization of the genitals may not reflect the degree of masculinization of the brain."

In other words, our sexual organs are differentiated *during* weeks six to twelve. The brain is sexually differentiated *after* this period. Because these two processes occur separately and can be subjected to different hormonal influences, genital masculinization does not necessarily correlate with the brain.

Drs. Swaab and Garcia-Falgueras are adamant: biology is the determinant. They disagree that social conditions influence gender identity. They note in young children, as well as in vervet and rhesus monkeys, gender-differentiated behavior in toy preference is seen as early as three months.

"There is no proof that social environment after birth has an effect on gender identity," say the scientists. "The changes brought about in this stage are permanent."

If you are beginning to get the feeling that more youths than ever are gender fluid, nonbinary, gender nonconforming, or identifying as transgender, you're right. It's undeniable. Fueled by Gen Z and the Millennials, the percentage of Americans identifying as LGBTQ+ increased from 3.5 percent in 2012 to 5.6 percent in 2020. That's almost double in just eight years when Gallup began tracking, based on over three hundred thousand interviews. Facebook, with nearly three billion users, has more than fifty gender identification options.[5, 6] Though many progressive local governments across the country are passing laws to identify bathrooms as gender neutral or "all-gender," other, less enlightened legislatures are passing harsh laws that discriminate against the LGBTQ+ community.[7, 8, 9]

No wonder, then, the number of adolescents contacting specialized gender-identity services across North America and Europe has risen over the past decade.[10]

Yes, of course, Facebook has more than fifty different shades of gender. But there's still way too much darkness.

Parents and so many elected officials, who don't know the science, need to learn how the gender dots are connected.

Total enlightenment hasn't brightened our society—at least not yet. Informed, educated parents play the pivotal role in their child's health. They must shine their light so their kids (or uneducated members of our society) won't be lost in the dark.

## Joy of Gender—A Family Protection Plan

The fetal or infant's developing brain is not a monolith of male or female carved in stone and never to be changed. A child's brain is plastic and gathering information from their internal and external environments. One thing we now know is that different regions of the fast-developing child's brain may be impacted as embryo, fetus, and in infancy by seemingly infinite chemical combinations, their amount, duration, and period of exposure.

We all contain attributes of both sexes. But gender identity generally has been polarized by religious, societal, and cultural demands that have been in complete opposition to how we *actually* feel inside. In reality, since the advent of the Kinsey scale in 1948, we've known sexual orientation and, more recently, gender identification, exist without formal or rigid definitions but, rather, on a continuum.[11] Gender identity is no longer a binary choice. It never was. Most of us just didn't know it.

Perhaps, instead of judging others, including our own children, we can become educated, helpful, and emotionally affirming. This is the positive action step we can take to help our kids, who are on their own journey, to become their authentic selves.

## *Trans or Gender Fluid?*

The general rule for determining whether a child is transgender or nonbinary (rather than gender nonconforming or gender variant) is if they're consistent, insistent, and persistent about their choice of identity, explains the Human Rights Campaign (HRC), a nonprofit group dedicated to advocacy on behalf of the LGBTQ+ community.

"In other words, if your four-year-old son wants to wear a dress or says he wants to be a girl once or twice, he probably is not transgender; but if your child who was assigned male at birth repeatedly insists over the course of several months or years, she is a girl, she is probably transgender."

Children won't necessarily have the vocabulary to articulate what they're feeling inside. But they will show you who they are through their actions and how they present or express themselves to society.

## *Identity or Orientation?*

Gender identity is not the same as sexual orientation.

Each of us has a gender identity and a sexual orientation. A person who identifies as transgender can also have a gay, lesbian, or bisexual orientation. Gender is about *identity* rather than *attraction*.

## *How to Support LGBTQ+ Kids*

Every professional whom I've interviewed has told me to share with parents the two things that count the most in raising healthy kids: Love first. Then educate.

(Very often, transgender-identifying children educate their parents.) The foundation of support is unconditional love and acceptance. Parents need to accept and love their kids unconditionally when and if they come out or otherwise identify themselves as different. Love first. Then become educated.

Judging, punishing, and denying won't work. Reparative and conversion therapy are harmful, say psychological, psychiatric, and medical organizations.[12]

No matter at what age, if your child comes out, they need to know you fiercely have their back, especially if push comes to shove and they are bullied and discriminated against at school or in other social situations.

The HRC recommends the following ways to support your transgender or nonbinary child:

- Always use the name and pronouns that align with your child's gender identity. Deadnaming (using the name of the transgender child assigned at birth) is harmful.
- Be your child's advocate—call out transphobia when you see it and ask others to respect your child's identity.
- Educate yourself about the concerns facing transgender youth and adults.
- Learn what schools can and should do to support and affirm your child.
- Encourage your child to stand up for themselves when it is safe to do so; to set boundaries when necessary; and to alert others if a situation becomes harmful or abusive.
- Assure your child they have your unconditional love and support, and you will be there for them.

## *The Turbulence of Gender Dysphoria*

Dana Beyer, MD, knows all about the impact of chemical toxins on gender identity as the adult child of a mother given the first of the synthetic fake estrogens, diethylstilbestrol (DES), during pregnancy. The drug was prescribed to millions of women in the United States and Europe, and it clearly causes gender dysphoria in their offspring (besides multigenerational cases of cancer).

Dr. Beyer, who identifies as transgender, has used her professional and personal knowledge and experience to change medicine's fundamental perception of the transgender experience by working with the American Psychiatric Association

(APA) to remove the medical stigma of identifying as transgender, changing its classification from a disease to a condition.

In the past, the turbulence kids and adults experienced in transitioning was classified as "gender identity disorder." Through her and others' efforts, however, in 2013, the diagnosis was changed. It became less ominous and more like a condition. "Gender dysphoria" became the new diagnosis when the APA's *Diagnostic and Statistical Manual of Mental Disorders* (DSM)-5 was published that year.[13, 14]

"Dysphoria means significant uneasiness when one's own internal sense of gender identity doesn't match their genitalia or gender they were assigned at birth," said Dr. Beyer. "But it's a condition one experiences for good reason in this society. It certainly isn't a disease."

In her own case, Dr. Beyer's earliest childhood memories from the age of six are when she began recognizing herself as a girl.

"I just knew who I was in my being," she told me confidently. "You can read Heidegger to get a philosophical sense of what that means. It's not a feeling; it's not gender nonconformity—you just know who you are."

Dr. Beyer came out at eleven when she began painting her nails. Her parents insisted she use the gender assigned to her at birth. She recalled having to sneak into bookstores in New York City to learn about what it was to identify as transgender.

After completing transitioning, long after becoming a physician who had performed thousands of eye surgeries, some in Africa where people were escaping genocide, as well as many more over a long career in the United States, Dr. Beyer's parents were serious when they asked her if she would continue to retain her license to practice medicine.

"There was a lot of ignorance out there," she said. "I had to live with it and do my best."

The diagnosis of "gender dysphoria" by a qualified doctor or therapist, however, has tremendous medical and insurance value. It can be the only way to have coverage for gender-affirming care that allows people to live their most authentic selves, added Dr. Beyer.

Gender therapy is for anyone questioning how they identify or who wants to develop a deeper understanding of themselves as they begin their own heroic journey.

A gender therapist is essential when medical interventions are undertaken, including treatments using puberty and testosterone blockers, estrogen, and testosterone, as well as chest, lower body, vocal cord, facial, tracheal, and body-contouring surgeries.

However, someone advertising themselves as a gender specialist, who is accepting of LGBTQ+ people, doesn't mean they are qualified, Mere advised.

"They should have a history of working with trans, nonbinary, gender nonconforming, or questioning persons," Mere added.

For kids who are questioning, finding the right therapists can be a valuable source of guidance that will pay healthy dividends and make their lives much easier.

The American Civil Liberties Union (ACLU) is tracking 452 pending anti-LGBTQ laws, most aimed at trans-identifying people, introduced in the United States in 2023.[15] That number continues to increase.[16]

In America, Europe, Russia, and elsewhere, when transgender acceptance is low and appropriate public facilities and health services aren't available, too many bright teens and youths end up contemplating and even committing suicide, harming themselves with drugs, or entering the illegal sex trade. They do this to acquire the funds to afford their medical treatments, because of social and family rejection, or both.

Taking away basic gender-affirming health care rights, targeting drag performers, and restricting access to public facilities hurts our children and is a retreat into a world of darkness. Legislation involving health care should reflect who we are today as a society, based on the best science and not superstition, or on who all of us were half a century and countless fake estrogen exposures ago.

Before Dr. Guillette passed away in 2015, he confessed the gators of Lake Apopka were in no better shape than when he had first begun studying them thirty years earlier.

Like the gators of Lake Apopka, our kids are swimming in a sea of estrogen. This is the new world. It's different today. Finding safe land can be difficult. Unconditional love and acceptance are their islands.

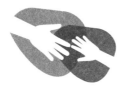

# Chapter 15

# The Power of Deep Caring

Anaïs (named for the powerful, self-assured writer Anaïs Nin) Peterson, aged fifteen, was entering a new high school in 2014 when their family moved from the suburbs of Chicago to surburban O'Hara Township, thirty miles east of Pittsburgh, Pennsylvania. Their father, Robert Nishikawa, a researcher in mammography, was about to take a faculty position at the University of Pittsburgh.

The hills and vales along the Allegheny River have a tragic history of catastrophic industrialism. Andrew Carnegie started his steel company, and other industry magnates brought their coke furnaces and zinc works to the shores of the Monongahela River, in the early 1900s. The plants are said to have operated twenty-four hours a day, seven days a week.

My family is from here. My mother Rose and other relatives hailed from Beaver Falls, Pennsylvania. People who remembered those times told me they could distinguish the zinc plants (that produced the metal needed to prevent corrosion of steel and iron) by the distinct lemon-colored clouds drifting from their smokestacks through the grassy dales of the rolling hills.[1]

Some of the older folks experienced those horrific five days that began before Halloween in late October 1948. Warm air floated above a lower, cooler layer to form a cap of motionless, yellow-black fog over the town of Donora and Webster hamlet.

Pets and plants died first, twenty-six people in all, another 5,900 (43 percent of the city's population) were sickened.

Donora's five-day killer fog was the first pollution-related tragedy that awakened the nation to the toxic poisoning of its land, water, and air.[2]

Seven decades after the event in Donora, Anaïs, a self-described "queer, mixed race Asian American prose poet, lyric essayist, and organizer," gazed up with wondering eyes at the brown haze that hovered from the remaining industrial plants of an older era—and an entirely new beast on the landscape: gas wells drilling Mother Earth to cash in on the Marcellus shale fracking boom.

They were going up everywhere, even nearby schools, and her family now realized they had moved to fracking country. Fracking wells and all of the needed infrastructure were going up everywhere in the surrounding area, even frighteningly close to schools, playgrounds, daycare centers, parks, and people's homes.

The rigs for the natural gas wells dotting the landscape rose up into the sky. They burned bright in the night.

They smelled like rotten eggs, gave people headaches, and hurt their lungs and eyes.

One proposed well especially concerned the family. This one was to be built near their home, all too close to a large park (complete with trails, ball fields, and streams where children play and people fish), daycare and elderly care facilities, and the soccer field where their younger brother, Boomba, played and Robert coached.[3, 4]

They talked about the situation, like they always did, at the dinner table, in the kitchen, on nightly walks in the woods, and with friends and neighbors. Dianne, Bob, and another concerned resident formed a local group to begin community education, raise public awareness, and generate support against the project. As they had done before the county council in their past efforts to keep fracking out of their parks, the family again testified—this time before the local township council. So did others in the community. But despite their efforts, they lost and this well and others all across their region kept getting permitted. Portions of their local park, named for the environmentalist Rachel Carson, were even relocated to accommodate the new fracking operation.

"The sad irony of it all!" Dianne exclaimed. "Even though we knew the well was coming, still, it was pretty shocking when we saw it one day as the backdrop of my son's soccer games."

But they didn't give up.

Anaïs learned activist groups like Zero Hour, 350.org, and NextGenAmerica. org were planning a march in Washington, DC and throughout the nation on July 21, 2018 to bring public awareness to the issue of climate change and the damaging impact of activities such as fracking.

"I realized no one was doing anything like that in Pittsburgh, so I said, 'I should get on that,'" Anaïs remembered.[5]

That day, seventy powerful activists, including Dianne, Bob, and Boomba, joined Anaïs, marching down Grant Street, in Pittsburgh, to the City-County Building to make their voices heard and take their message of a fossil fuel–free future directly to state and federal politicians.

Anaïs spoke to the crowd and demanded an end to fracking in Allegheny County.

The powerful mother-child duo took part in more demonstrations. They dressed up as petro zombies for one of them, the Shale Insight conference in Pittsburgh. Anaïs wore makeup with blood everywhere over their face and a grotesque-looking fake wound visible through a tear in their shirt. An older white male fracking executive walking into the conference social event passed them by. He seemingly ignored the point of the protest and instead noticed Anaïs and their bare midriff, making a lewd, misogynistic comment as he passed by them inside.[6]

Eight years after drilling operations began in Allegheny County, at Deer Lakes Park near Tarentum, Anaïs and their family were back at it, among protesters gathered on the steps of the City-County Building in downtown Pittsburgh ahead of a June 9, 2022, public hearing. Anaïs spoke to rally support for a council bill that would prohibit hydraulic fracturing (also known as "hydrofracking") on any of the county's remaining potential sites.

"You have the choice to be brave . . . and do what is right," Anaïs told public officials.

The Allegheny County Council voted one month later, in July 2022, overwhelmingly to ban fracking in public parks. However, Allegheny County Executive Rich Fitzgerald—"much like an Hungarian autocrat thinking he knew better," said Dianne—vetoed the ban. But it wasn't over. Anaïs had an innovative and simple idea they used before in their activism efforts in college (leading the fight for the university to divest from fossil fuels). They named their action "Cookies for a Call." The superhero duo journeyed into town and began informing folks about the situation, asking they call their county council member, and giving them a cookie or other treat to snack on while they did.

With a vote of 12 to 3, the Allegheny County Council overrode Fitzgerald's veto for the first time ever in its history with him to allow the law go into effect.

After the vote, Dianne spoke with one of the council members she had fought with for eight years over fracking in county parks and asked why he changed his vote. He confirmed that Anaïs's "Cookie For a Call" strategy was a winner.

"I got so many damned calls from my constituents on this, I had to vote this way," he told Dianne.

I spoke with Dianne a few days after her mother, Dorothy, passed away at age ninety-six in January 2023. It was a time of reflection. At first, Dianne said she was overloaded, making funeral arrangements, had a lot on her mind, and needed time. She called me back fifteen minutes later and let loose a torrent of feelings and observations.

It was impossible to listen without pulling over to the side of the road along the green winter mountains of State Highway 27 in California. I grabbed my reporter's notebook and began writing, and it was tough, I have to say, to keep up with every important word she shared:

"I don't like to say how proud I am of what my children have become, as if I have 'created them,'" Dianne said. "I didn't create them! That's ridiculous. Whatever they've become is due to their own abilities, work, and effort. My husband and I provided for them, gave them opportunities, shared our thoughts, and, most important, cared about them. We deeply cared and still do.

"From the beginning of child-rearing, we worked hard to promote that each member of our family deeply care about each other. Deep caring means commitment. People ask how did we get so close as a family. We show up for each other. We made the effort to attend everything that each of us does: soccer games, band performances, debate competitions, marches, protests, talks, testifying before the state's Department of Environmental Protection, US Environmental Protection Agency, and various city and county boards and representatives. You name it. If one is involved, the rest of us will try our best to be there every time! We didn't tell my kids what they had to be. We loved them and supported them for whatever good they were doing, whatever issue they wanted to take on. As parents, we have always been mindful that diet and lifestyle continuously work to reduce our children's exposure to chemical toxins and plastics and, more and more, we pay attention to our indoor and outdoor air quality. I think it makes a big difference both because of the reduction in exposures and because they see how much their father and I care about them.

"I don't believe any person can care about an issue without first being deeply cared about. One learns to care both through the act of being cared for and by witnessing the act of caring firsthand. I was taught as a child to recycle and, more important, to be mindful not to waste and have done so for my entire life. I grew up in a home where my mom, Dorothy, who had a car only one day a week, would take the time that day to drive thirty minutes out of her way to make sure we recycled everything possible.

"I see my mother as both mother and grandmother to a family of activists. And I see it as both my honor and duty to have continued to help my mom speak out even after she was in a wheelchair and could no longer do so herself. We packed up my mom's handpainted signs and wheelchair and took her—at ninety-two years young—to the march in Washington for climate change. She was there. I was and so was Anaïs. We were together. Bob and Boomba, our entire family. We protest and do actions together.

"We would take the kids with us to testify. I've learned to testify. We need people to testify. We need people to take up a cause. It can be climate change. No more plastic. Anti-pesticides, whatever grabs you. It doesn't need to be in your backyard because, frankly, everyplace on Earth is someone's backyard, and *any* backyard is all of our backyards!

"I used to think these things happened someplace else, you know, over there, out of sight, but if they're not happening next to me, to you, to our kids, then it's happening to someone else and someone else's kids! It's so unfair how industry is changing our bodies, our kids' bodies, and the genetics for our children's future children and grandchildren with endocrine disruptors from plastics and toxins everywhere (in our land, water, and air). There's always something that needs to be done, so many causes that need our time to be worked on.

"We all say, 'We're busy and have no time.' Do folks really 'have no time'? Of course some folks truly don't have the time or energy. I understand some folks are already at capacity, for example by being caretakers or holding down multiple jobs to provide for their needs. And of course everyone should have a balance of free time in their lives, but if one has time enough to watch a television program or two every night then they probably have enough time to give at least a half hour a week to a cause! Frankly I don't even care if it's one of 'my causes,' because there are so many! Look around, keep your eyes and ears open, see what is happening locally, ask questions, do some research, join (or start) a local group, and, once you know enough, take action: inform your friends and neighbors; write a letter to the editor; call, write to, and meet with your representatives as many times as it takes. Throwing money at a cause or posting on social media is 'okay,' but there's so much more you can do that will have a larger impact. Get personally involved! Once you do, you will find joy in caring, in caring deeply, and maybe—just maybe—make a difference! If you want to make things better, you have to care. You have to care deeply. You have to care about this country and its people. None of us here in Allegheny County or anyplace else on the planet want to be part of a sacrifice zone."

## Deep Caring—A Family Protection Plan

As parents, grandparents, educators, and youth mentors, we have an opportunity to learn about the tools and experiences that can help shape kids into environmentally aware citizens.[7] We know how important a parent or mentor is to the process. Sharing nature at an early age is a powerful way to start your child on the path of environmental awareness.

### Help Your Child Experience Nature

The classic journey into environmental awareness is through nature. For Rachel Carson, growing up on a farm in rural Pennsylvania led to her work as a biologist near the seashore at Woods Hole and ultimately authoring her first book, *Under the Sea-Wind*. Hiking in the Arizona mountains led Stewart Udall to become, perhaps, our nation's greatest Secretary of the Department of Interior throughout the 1960s under two presidential administrations. As a child, Sharon C. Lavigne of St. James Parish in Louisiana used to to enjoy consuming the fish and shrimp her grandfather caught from the waters of the Mississippi River. Brenda Hampton remembers when she was a child and her beloved Tennessee River was world famous for its freshwater mussel populations. For my friend Oscar Ramos, it was coming within touching distance of the late Cesar Chavez and, of course, being a resident of a town made out of farm fields.

Joel Ussery, of Lincoln, California, who goes by @sustainajoel on social media, posted a video on TikTok of his young daughter Aspen's first time touching a pine needle.

"It's pokey," she said, recoiling, uttering no when Joel tried to have her touch another bough.

"It's fun . . . it's like a comb," Joel said, brushing a bough gently through her hair. "They're also soft," he added.

"They're not pokey?" she said, wondrously.

"With technology constantly at our fingertips, it's important to disconnect from tech and re-associate with the Earth," Joel wrote on his social media. "This is especially important for our children as they are growing up with more distractions [than] ever before. The garden, when planted organically, creates a space for us to associate with the Earth on a daily basis. The soil, plants, insects, animals, and trillions of microorganisms that congregate in a garden are the life that doesn't exist in the digital world. It is only in these spaces, whether wild or maintained, that we can quiet our minds, dig our hands into the soil, and remember how intimately connected we are to all of it."

But what if your home doesn't have space for a garden? Even a balcony or window with good sun is suitable to grow bountiful gardens of potted or raised-bed herbs, veggies, and fruits. It's fun when you take a little slice of strawberry, put it in moist soil, and a healthy baby bud with multiple vines and sprouts appear.

Rosemary, parsley, sage, mint, and oregano, available in pots at garden shops, are easy to grow on a balcony or windowsill. Dwarf mandarin and peach trees can also do well in many climate zones.

Community-supported agriculture (CSA) is not only a convenient and cost-effective way to buy organic foods and keep small community farms alive; participating helps children see the connection between their food on the table and where it comes from. Many CSA organizations are nonprofits designed to connect communities with local farms. They offer a weekly box of in-season produce for pick up or delivery.

Participants may pay weekly or buy seasonal shares, which affords the farm financial security. The US Department of Agriculture (USDA) CSA directory (https://www.ams.usda.gov/local-food-directories/csas) is the place to start to find a nearby farm or organization.[8]

Your local farmers' market is a powerful way to connect kids with where their food comes from. Plus, farmers' markets often have free tasting and better prices than a lot of supermarkets.

In cities such as Winston-Salem, New York, and Detroit, community gardens are an oasis in food deserts.[9] Garden members share a plot of land where they grow their own produce. The American Community Garden Association lists more than two thousand shared plots across the land. Visit them at https://www.communitygarden.org/.

Microgreens are one of the best activities for children when outdoor gardens aren't available. Microgreens, used with salads, sandwiches, or as snacks, are filled with healthy anti-cancer phytonutrients and mature quickly—usually in as short as one to three weeks—and are harvested when only one to three inches tall and their first true leaves appear. Popular microgreens kids can grow, and enjoy eating and learning about include beets, broccoli, cabbage, carrots, celery, cilantro, kale, lettuce, mustard greens, parsley, peas, radishes, and spinach. Microgreen kits are available online at Amazon.com.

## Down on the Farm

"Get a little dirty, have a lot of fun and teach your children that food doesn't come from the grocery store," states upickfarmlocator.com, an online directory of farms that invite you to pick your own fruits and veggies. The farm locator works by zip code and preferences. I used my zip and discovered several nearby cherry and apple farms.

Most farms and orchards are kid-friendly as they see the value of teaching children where their food comes from and to appreciate locally grown produce. Some offer wagon rides, petting zoos, corn mazes, and playgrounds.

## Plant Trees

"Let's plant trees!" says Greyson (Boo), son of Instagram influencer Addie Fisher (@oldworldnew), a sustainable living enthusiast. By the time Boo was five, he had already helped raise nearly nine hundred dollars to plant trees. Boo's birthdays have become a tree-planting bonanza, and every year Addie sets a goal for them to continue their mini-reforestation project.

Little Boo was turning six this year, and it was a time to plant more trees!

"Another chance to give back to Mama Earth and the people who are helping her to thrive again," Addie wrote.

Boo's goal in 2022 was to raise six hundred dollars for the global group treesforthefuture.org, which educates farming families across nine countries in sub-Saharan Africa in restorative agroforestry, repopulating barren landscapes.

The Arbor Day Foundation created the Community Tree Recovery program in 2005 out of the great need for trees in the Gulf Coast following Hurricane

Katrina. When you or your child join the Arbor Day Foundation, you will receive ten free trees to plant. The foundation is also helping get free trees into the hands of affected homeowners throughout the nation who've lost theirs due to disasters caused by wildfires, floods, hurricanes, tornadoes, and insects. Visit arborday.org to find out more.

## *Green Heroes*

Storytelling transforms self-perceptions and fortifies and charges up children to go out and protect the earth. Green literature for kids is a powerful genre featuring stories of diverse heroes who inspire, empower, and support environmentally aware children of all colors (whose caring for nature also makes them an inspiration to others).

*The New York Times* bestseller *We Are Water Protectors* by Carole Lindstrom, a member of the Turtle Mountain Band of Ojibwe, is for kids ages three to six. Lindstrom shares a story about the environmental activism of Indigenous peoples told from the perspective of a Native American girl.

*The Thing About Bees: A Love Letter* by Shabazz Larkin is a picture book for kids ages three to seven that can turn a child's fear of bees into wonder. The narrator of this empowering story is a Black beekeeper representing a community largely inhabited by white people.

*Arthur Turns Green* by Marc Brown, for kids ages six to nine, is about a boy whose class assignment is to find ways to make the Earth a better place and all of his discoveries as he learns how to care for our planet.

*Amara and the Bats* by Emma Reynolds, for ages four to eight, is about a girl who finds a bat in her attic and learns to care about them and how important they are to our ecology. But there were none any longer at the local park. Amara solicits family and friends to restore their original habitat.

*Follow the Moon Home* by Philippe Cousteau and Deborah Hopkinson is about a child who learns houselights in her new neighborhood are confusing the turtles hatching on the beach nearby where she lives. They head away from the water and die. Once again, an individual voice helps to win the day by organizing the town so that the lights go dark, and baby turtles can find their way to the sea.

As kids get older, they will want to connect online. Green websites bring together kids, tweens, and teens around the world to learn, share ideas, tell their stories, and develop the practical skills that will allow them to meet the challenges of personal, local, national, and global environmental issues in a safe, mentored space.

Earthforce.org is for middle and high school tweens and teens. Its Young Executive program develops skills to lead environmental actions and spread the word about the need to live more sustainable lifestyles. Kids come up with solutions to local issues. In Wentzville, Missouri, persons living in multiple-family units had to drive to recycling centers. The Earthforce teens partnered with local government and homeowner associations to create an onsite recycling program for them.

TurningGreen.org is one of my favorite organizations. Their website is a transformative destination for teens and college students who want to know how to make smart shopping choices that positively impact their health and our environment. TurningGreen offers eco-themed challenges for college dorms, home, kitchen, school, and personal care and beauty products with guidance on conscious living, informed consumption, individual, and collective action.

Youth4Nature.org is an international nonprofit organization that educates, empowers, and mobilizes teens to collaborate on solutions for the ecological and climate crises rooted in science, aligned with indigenous knowledge, and grounded in environmental justice. Their mission is to elevate the voices of young people by providing a platform to share their stories and have them be heard—and build a youth movement as stewards for nature and climate.

Jacqueline Ellis, twenty-three, of Chattanooga, Tennessee, found growing up in the South, together with her mixed Asian heritage, could be "kind of a strange" experience.[10] She gained confidence as assistant leader for an all-women's crew with the Southeast Conservation Corps.

"Everyone has a place on the crew," she said. "It doesn't matter where you're from or experience level. When you work with a bunch of dudes, unfortunately, as a woman you feel like you have to prove yourself. Coming into this and working with a crew of women is a safe place and not as intimidating. In the beginning I was really apprehensive about doing stuff because I wasn't comfortable just getting in there and doing it. Here, you go in. You make a mistake. But it's not the end of the world. That is definitely something I am going to take from this experience and apply to other jobs."

With their office in Chattanooga, nestled between the Cumberland Plateau and the Appalachian Mountains, the Southeast Conservation Corps engages a diverse population of youths in a broad range of conservation service projects and recreation opportunities within some of the oldest and most biologically diverse forests in the eastern United States.

The United States has some 108 service corps programs operating in 200 communities across 31 states and the District of Columbia. Corps are organizations that engage young adults (generally ages sixteen to thirty) and veterans (up to age thirty-five) in service projects that address local conservation and community needs. Participants are compensated with a stipend or living allowance and often receive an education award or scholarship upon completing their service.

Volunteering to work in nature with other youth can become a powerful experience in a teen's life and an ideal way to spend some of their summertime. Visit Corpsnetwork.org to find a local state or nonprofit organization.

The federal Youth Conservation Corps (YCC), a summer employment program, engages young people from fifteen to thirty in meaningful work experiences at national parks, forests, wildlife refuges, and fish hatcheries.

Enrollment begins in February through April 15. Visit https://www.nps.gov/subjects/youthprograms/ycc.htm.

We didn't even have the language of environmentalism until sixty years ago when Rachel Carson wrote *Silent Spring*. None of us could have imagined concepts such as one part per million, billion, or trillion, endocrine disruptors, or fake estrogens. No one had ever heard of an environmental impact report or law that would give citizens the power to fight pollution. Conservation, or, what then passed for environmentalism, involved preserving mountains, seashores, and rivers, and stopping dams. No one knew a thing about Teflon, organic agriculture, or toxic exposures that rewired children's brains. Sure, a few informed citizens and scientists knew, but not the people. But now we do. We need to continue our studies to understand things better. But we know enough to take action to protect our families and communities. For that, we don't need more studies. We need to be able to count on each other and our elected officials.

Nature is the starting point to creating environmentally sensitive, healthy children. Nature can even heal children with attention deficit/hyperactivity disorder.[11]

But, along with nature, kids need to see your activism. Is your local council considering permitting a fracking well? Protest! Is there a cell phone tower being considered close to a nearby park? March! Is your school district considering building a school on a brownfield? Testify! Is your council about to vote on housing or school that would be built on or nearby where there is coal ash? Write an editorial for your local paper!

Let your kids see you take action.

Get out there. Do something. Go local or global. Demonstrate. Groups like 350.org, Sunrise Movement, Extinction Rebellion, and Sierra Club can alert you to events in your area and would love to have your family's support.

Help your child write a letter to their representative, prepare to testify, or even form a community-action group. Show them they can be heard and their voice and views count.

It's not difficult to write a compelling letter to your member of Congress, state house, local city or county government. The same model can also be used if your child would like to offer public testimony.

Here's a basic outline:

**Introduce yourself.** Share something personal. Tell the representative your age, where you live, and the school you attend.

**Share your concern.** Tell the official why the issue is important personally and to the community. If it's too much trash at the local park, describe the situation. If it's about permitting yet another plastics plant, mention its toxic impact on the local environment. Maybe it's a matter of creating safe passages for wildlife to cross busy roadways. There will be no shortage of local health issues needing your child's voice.

**Make the ask.** Showing kids they have agency empowers them. Teaching them how to ask for what is needed is part of civics 101 and makes them more capable in all areas of their lives. They can say, "This is why I want you to support [cosponsor/oppose and name the bill or project]."

**Conclude.** Thank your representative and state that you look forward to their response.

I promised to shine light. The steps I've shared are as simple as A-B-C. But they will do so much to keep your children safe.

It's important to recognize our personal shopping choices also hold enormous power.

We're winning.

We just need to take a moment to reflect on how far we've come.

Who created the organic market?

We did.

Who created the market for safe beauty products?

It was us.

How about the green cleaning product industry?

Look in the mirror.

Every shopping choice we make has a vital local impact. I saw this when I witnessed acts in Salinas, California, that confirmed my faith that the actions we take really do make a positive difference.

The more of us who become smart shoppers, the fewer harmful chemicals will be demanded. This will help to push the politicians toward passing tough laws that demand public disclosure of carcinogens and reproductive toxins before we buy products, allow citizen enforcement, and impose stiff civil penalties for violations.

This is how I see things: through the lens of an activist and citizen enforcer, but most of all as a parent to my kids.

Be the role model your kids need. Be the love and acceptance they crave.

Let them see you commit to activism at home, when shopping, and in public. You can be quiet and work behind the scenes, testify before the county board of supervisors, or carry a sign and march. Most of all, make it personal. There are so many different ways of deep caring.

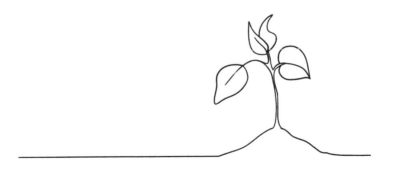

# Appendix

## CR REVEALS: | WHO HAS PFAS IN THEIR FOOD WRAPPERS?

THESE RESULTS SHOW levels of total organic fluorine, a measure of PFAS, in 118 food packaging products gathered from major fast-food and fast-casual restaurants, as well as supermarkets. PFAS in food

| Arby's | | PPM |
|---|---|---|
| Bag for cookies | ■ ■ | 457.5 |
| Wrapper for sandwich wrap | ■ | 32.0 |
| Wrapper for Classic Roast Beef sandwich | | 12.0 |
| Wrapper for Classic Beef 'N Cheddar sandwich | | 8.5 |
| Container for french fries | | ND |
| Container for sliders | | ND |

| Burger King | | |
|---|---|---|
| Bag for cookies, French toast sticks | ■ ■ | 345.7 |
| Wrapper for Whopper | ■ ■ | 249.7 |
| Bag for chicken nuggets | ■ ■ | 165.0 |
| Container for french fries | | 13.0 |
| Container for chicken, french fries | | 12.0 |
| Container for tater tots | | 8.5 |

| Cava | | |
|---|---|---|
| Fiber tray for kids meal | ■ ■ | 548.0 |
| Fiber bowl for grains, salad | ■ ■ | 508.3 |
| Wrapper for mini pita, pita sandwich | ■ ■ | 280.0 |
| Bag for pita chips | ■ ■ | 260.0 |
| Wrapper for pita | ■ ■ | 202.0 |
| Wrapper for sides | | 13.3 |

| Checkers | | |
|---|---|---|
| Container for french fries | ■ | 27.0 |
| Wrapper for chicken, hamburger | | 15.0 |
| Container for chili dog | | ND |
| Container for chicken bites with french fries | | ND |

| Chick-fil-A | | PPM |
|---|---|---|
| Wrapper for sandwich wrap | ■ ■ | 553.5 |
| Bag for sandwich FOIL-LINED | | 10.5 |
| Container for sides | | 8.5 |

| Chipotle | | |
|---|---|---|
| Fiber bowl with four compartments | ■ | 35.5 |
| Wrapper for burrito | ■ | 26.3 |
| Fiber bowl for sides, meals | | 11.7 |

| Five Guys | | |
|---|---|---|
| Wrapper for hamburger ALUMINUM FOIL | | 8.0 |
| Container for french fries | | ND |
| Wrapper for vegetable sandwich ALUMINUM FOIL | | ND |
| Wrapper for hot dog ALUMINUM FOIL | | ND |

| Freshii | | |
|---|---|---|
| Fiber bowl for salad | | 16.7 |
| Wrapper for burrito, wrap | | 9.7 |

| Hannaford | | |
|---|---|---|
| Bakery plate under cake | ■ | 23.3 |
| Baking nonstick aluminum foil | | ND |
| Paper plates GREASE-RESISTANT | | ND |
| Bakery sheet | | ND |

| Kroger | | PPM |
|---|---|---|
| Baking cups | ■ | 51.3 |
| Tray for take-and-bake double pepperoni pizza | | 15.0 |
| Paper plates GREASE-RESISTANT | | ND |
| Baking liner for muffins | | ND |

| McDonald's | | |
|---|---|---|
| Bag for french fries | ■ ■ | 250.3 |
| Bag for cookies | ■ ■ | 250.0 |
| Bag for Chicken McNuggets | ■ ■ | 219.0 |
| Container for Big Mac | ■ ■ | 195.3 |
| Wrapper for double cheeseburger | | 15.0 |
| Container for Chicken McNuggets | | 13.5 |
| Container for french fries | | 7.5 |
| Wrapper for Egg McMuffin | | 7.0 |
| Wrapper for McChicken sandwich | | ND |

| Nathan's Famous | | |
|---|---|---|
| Bag for sides GREEN STRIPE | ■ ■ | 876.0 |
| Bag for sides RED STRIPE | ■ ■ | 618.0 |
| Wrapper for sandwich | ■ ■ | 104.0 |
| Container for hamburger | ■ | 42.0 |
| Container for hot dog | | 9.8 |
| Container for fish sandwich | | ND |
| Container for french fries | | ND |
| Container for shrimp sandwich | | ND |

**Note:** Products were selected based on availability at the time of the visit (August to November 2021) at stores in Connecticut, Mississippi, New Jersey, New York, and Texas. Levels shown are averages of multiple samples of each product. All packaging is paper-based unless otherwise noted. Results are not representative of all the packaging from a retailer, and packaging may have changed since CR conducted these tests. "ND" means "not detected" (the test, which can generally detect 10 ppm or more, did not find any organic fluorine).

packaging have been linked to potential harms to human health and the environment. Products with two squares have 100 parts per million organic fluorine or more. Starting next year, California will ban food packaging that exceeds that level. Products with one square have 20 ppm organic fluorine or more, a stricter standard for food packaging set by Denmark. CR supports that lower cutoff.

**Key**

| | |
|---|---|
| ■ | 20 PPM OR MORE |
| ■ ■ | 100 PPM OR MORE |
| ND | NOT DETECTED |

## Panera Bread

| | | PPM |
|---|---|---|
| Container for flatbread pizza | ■ | 82.0 |
| Bag for baguette | ■ | 35.7 |
| Wrapper for sandwich | ■ | 30.3 |

## Popeyes

| | PPM |
|---|---|
| Bag for french fries | 9.3 |
| Bag for sandwich<br>FOIL-LINED | 7.0 |

## Roy Rogers

| | | |
|---|---|---|
| Wrapper for hamburger<br>FOIL-LINED | ■ | 29.0 |
| Container for french fries | | 12.5 |
| Wrapper for breakfast sandwich | | 10.5 |
| Container for baked beans | | 8.0 |

## Shake Shack

| | |
|---|---|
| Container for hamburger | 10.5 |
| Container for hot dog | 10.3 |
| Container for french fries | 8.3 |
| Container for chicken nuggets | 7.0 |

## Smashburger

| | |
|---|---|
| Wrapper for breakfast sandwich | 9.5 |
| Container for french fries | ND |
| Wrapper for hamburger | ND |

## Stop & Shop

| | | |
|---|---|---|
| Paper plates<br>BAMBOO | ■ ■ | 368.7 |
| Paper plates<br>GREASE-RESISTANT | ■ ■ | 226.7 |
| Tray for store-brand thin-crust extra cheese pizza | ■ | 23.0 |

## Stop & Shop *continued*

| | | PPM |
|---|---|---|
| Baking cups<br>PASTEL | ■ | 22.0 |
| Bakery tray under cake<br>ROUND | | 12.0 |
| Wrapper for unsalted butter | | ND |
| Bakery tray under cake<br>RECTANGULAR | | ND |
| Bakery box for bakery items | | ND |
| Baking cups<br>PARTY DESIGN | | ND |
| Wrapper for sandwich | | ND |
| Bakery sheet | | ND |
| Bakery cup for muffin | | ND |

## Sweetgreen

| | | |
|---|---|---|
| Paper bag for focaccia | ■ ■ | 288.0 |
| Fiber bowl for salad | | 9.3 |
| Fiber bowl for sides, meals | | 8.8 |

## Taco Bell

| | | |
|---|---|---|
| Paper bag for chips | ■ ■ | 145.0 |
| Wrapper for taco | | 10.0 |
| Wrapper for burrito | | 9.3 |
| Takeout container for Chicken Power Bowl<br>PLASTIC | | ND |

## Trader Joe's

| | | |
|---|---|---|
| Bakery box for pancake bread | ■ ■ | 167.0 |
| Bakery tray under Patisserie de Chocolat cake | | 12.5 |
| Bowl for frozen chicken pot pie | | 10.5 |

## Trader Joe's *continued*

| | PPM |
|---|---|
| Bakery cups for chocolate chip muffins | ND |
| Wrapper for unsalted butter | ND |
| Wrapper for cultured salted butter | ND |
| Tray for frozen 5 Cheese Greek Spiral | ND |

## Wendy's

| | |
|---|---|
| Wrapper for hamburger | 16.7 |
| Paper bag for cookies | 10.3 |
| Container for french fries, chicken nuggets<br>JUNIOR | ND |
| Container for french fries, chicken nuggets<br>MEDIUM | ND |

## White Castle

| | | |
|---|---|---|
| Container for clam strips | ■ | 26.0 |
| Container for hamburger | | 14.0 |
| Container for sides<br>SMALL | | ND |
| Container for sides<br>MEDIUM | | ND |
| Container for fried sides | | ND |

## Whole Foods Market

| | | |
|---|---|---|
| Container for soup | ■ | 21.0 |
| Wrapper for salted butter | | 15.0 |
| Takeout container | | 14.0 |
| Bakery plate under cake | | 13.3 |
| Bakery parchment paper, 365 Whole Foods Market brand | | 13.0 |
| Wrapper for sandwich | | 12.2 |
| Bakery cup for muffin | | ND |
| Bakery sheet | | ND |

Used with permission of *Consumer Reports* Copyright © 2023. All rights reserved.

# Endnotes

### Introduction

1 Francis, L., DePriest, K., Wilson, M., & Gross, D. (2018). "Child Poverty, Toxic Stress, and Social Determinants of Health: Screening and Care Coordination." *Online journal of issues in nursing, 23*(3), 2. https://doi.org/10.3912/OJIN.Vol23No03Man02.

2 David Steinman and the Chemical Toxin Working Group, Inc vs. Chicken of the Sea International; Tri-Union Seafoods, LLC d/b/a Chicken of the Sea International; Bumble Bee Foods, LLC and DOES 1-100, Superior Court of the State of California County of Marin, Case No. CIV 1202604, June 27, 2012, https://oag.ca.gov/system/files/prop65/settlements/2012-00104S3250.pdf.

3 Office of the Attorney General 60 Day Notice 2015-00979, The Chemical Toxin Working Group, Inc. v. Tri-Union Seafoods, LLC d/b/a Chicken of the Seas International, https://oag.ca.gov/prop65/60-Day-Notice-2015-00979.

4 David Steinman v. The Procter and Gamble Distributing LLC Consent Judgement, Superior Court of the State of California County of San Francisco, Case No. CGC-10-500758, July 30, 2010, https://oag.ca.gov/system/files/prop65/judgments/2010-00119J1103.pdf.

5 David Steinman and the Chemical Toxin Working Group, Inc., a California non-profit corporation, v. Crown Prince, Inc. and DOES 1-100, Defendants, Coordinated Proceedings Special Title (rule 3.550) Proposition 65 Canned Food Cases and Coordinated Action, Judicial Council Coordination Proceeding No. 4779/Alameda County Case Nos. RG 13673501 and RG 13699240, https://oag.ca.gov/system/files/prop65/settlements/2012-00006S4560.pdf.

6 Office of the Attorney General 60 Day Notice 2021-01049, The Chemical Toxin Working Group Inc. v. Patagonia, https://oag.ca.gov/prop65/60-Day-Notice-2021-01049.

7 National Academy of Sciences, "Multiple Chemical Sensitivities: A Workshop," Washington, D.C.: National Academies Press (US), 1992.

8 Pell, T., Eliot, M., Chen, A., Lanphear, B. P., Yolton, K., Sathyanarayana, S., & Braun, J. M. (2017). "Parental Concern about Environmental Chemical Exposures and Children's Urinary Concentrations of Phthalates and Phenols." *The Journal of Pediatrics, 186*, 138–144.e3. https://doi.org/10.1016/j.jpeds.2017.03.064.

## Chapter 1

1 Environmental Protection Agency, "Research Centers, UC Berkeley School of Public Health: CHAMACOS Office, Berkeley, CAm https://cfpub.epa.gov/ncer_abstracts/index.cfm/fuseaction/outlinks.centers/center/191.

2 Gunier, R. B., Bradman, A., Harley, K. G., Kogut, K., & Eskenazi, B. (2017). "Prenatal Residential Proximity to Agricultural Pesticide Use and IQ in 7-Year-Old Children." *Environmental Health Perspectives, 125*(5), 057002. https://doi.org/10.1289/EHP504.

3 Marks, A. R., Harley, K., Bradman, A., Kogut, K., Barr, D. B., Johnson, C., Calderon, N., & Eskenazi, B. (2010). "Organophosphate pesticide exposure and attention in young Mexican-American children: the CHAMACOS study." *Environmental health Perspectives, 118*(12), 1768–1774. https://doi.org/10.1289/ehp.1002056.

4 Sagiv, S. K., Bruno, J. L., Baker, J. M., Palzes, V., Kogut, K., Rauch, S., Gunier, R., Mora, A. M., Reiss, A. L., & Eskenazi, B. (2019). "Prenatal exposure to organophosphate pesticides and functional neuroimaging in adolescents living in proximity to pesticide application." *Proceedings of the National Academy of Sciences of the United States of America, 116*(37), 18347–18356. https://doi.org/10.1073/pnas.1903940116.

5 Rauh, V. A., Garfinkel, R., Perera, F. P., Andrews, H. F., Hoepner, L., Barr, D. B., Whitehead, R., Tang, D., & Whyatt, R. W. (2006). "Impact of prenatal chlorpyrifos exposure on neurodevelopment in the first 3 years of life among inner-city children." *Pediatrics, 118*(6), e1845–e1859. https://doi.org/10.1542/peds.2006-0338.

6 Rauh, V., Arunajadai, S., Horton, M., Perera, F., Hoepner, L., Barr, D. B., & Whyatt, R. (2011). "Seven-year neurodevelopmental scores and prenatal exposure to chlorpyrifos, a common agricultural pesticide." *Environmental Health Perspectives, 119*(8), 1196–1201. https://doi.org/10.1289/ehp.1003160.

7 "Pesticide Residue Monitoring Program Fiscal Year 2020 Pesticide Report," U.S. Food and Drug Administration. https://www.fda.gov/media/160464/download?utm_medium=email&utm_source=govdelivery.

8 "Annual Residue Data, Pesticide Residue Monitoring Program," California Department of Pesticide Regulation, 2015–2020. https://www.cdpr.ca.gov/docs/enforce/residue/rsmonmnu.htm.

9 Lu, C., Toepel, K., Irish, R., Fenske, R. A., Barr, D. B., & Bravo, R. (2006). "Organic diets significantly lower children's dietary exposure to organophosphorus pesticides." *Environmental Health Perspectives, 114*(2), 260–263. https://doi.org/10.1289/ehp.8418.

10 Fagan, J., Bohlen, L., Patton, S., & Klein, K. (2020). "Organic diet intervention significantly reduces urinary glyphosate levels in U.S. children and adults." *Environmental Research, 189*, 109898. https://doi.org/10.1016/j.envres.2020.109898.

11 Hyland, C., Bradman, A., Gerona, R., Patton, S., Zakharevich, I., Gunier, R. B., & Klein, K. (2019). "Organic diet intervention significantly reduces urinary pesticide levels in U.S. children and adults." *Environmental Research, 171*, 568–575. https://doi.org/10.1016/j.envres.2019.01.024.

12  Curl, C. L., Porter, J., Penwell, I., Phinney, R., Ospina, M., & Calafat, A. M. (2019). "Effect of a 24-week randomized trial of an organic produce intervention on pyrethroid and organophosphate pesticide exposure among pregnant women." *Environment International*, *132*, 104957. https://doi.org/10.1016/j.envint.2019.104957.

13  Kazimierczak, R., Średnicka-Tober, D., Golba, J., Nowacka, A., Hołodyńska-Kulas, A., Kopczyńska, K., Góralska-Walczak, R., & Gnusowski, B. (2022). "Evaluation of Pesticide Residues Occurrence in Random Samples of Organic Fruits and Vegetables Marketed in Poland." *Foods (Basel, Switzerland)*, *11*(13), 1963. https://doi .org/10.3390/foods11131963.

14  US Food and Drug Administration—Total Diet Study Market Baskets 1991-3 through 2003-4.

15  Cao, F., Martyniuk, C. J., Wu, P., Zhao, F., Pang, S., Wang, C., & Qiu, L. (2019). "Long-Term Exposure to Environmental Concentrations of Azoxystrobin Delays Sexual Development and Alters Reproduction in Zebrafish (Danio rerio)." *Environmental Science & Technology*, *53*(3), 1672–1679. https://doi.org/10.1021/acs .est.8b05829.

16  Chakravorty, A. "Study finds washing effectively removes lead from vegetables grown in urban soil," Phys.org, August 23, 2022. https://phys.org/news/2022-08-effectively -vegetables-grown-urban-soil.html.

17  Egendorf, S. P., Li, E., He, E., Cheng, Z., Spliethoff, H. M., Shayler, H. A., Russell-Anelli, J., King, T., & McBride, M. B. (2022). "Effectiveness of washing in reducing lead concentrations of lettuce grown in urban garden soils." *Journal of Environmental Quality*, *51*(4), 755–764. https://doi.org/10.1002/jeq2.20357.

18  Caldwell, M. "Salinas grade school sits in a field where Diazinon and other pesticides are sprayed. Schoolyard Chemical Drift," *Monterey County Now*, May 27, 2004, updated May 17, 2013. https://www.montereycountyweekly.com/news/local_news/ salinas-grade-school-sits-in-a-field-where-diazinon-and-other-pesticides-are-sprayed/ article_09d9ae5a-5013-520f-b4b5-80ac072c66db.html.

## Chapter 2

1  Chen, H., Liang, X., Chen, L., Zuo, L., Chen, K., Wei, Y., Chen, S., & Hao, G. (2022). "Associations Between Household Pesticide Exposure, Smoking and Hypertension." *Frontiers in Public Health*, *10*, 754643. https://doi.org/10.3389/fpubh.2022.754643.

2  Goncharov, A., Pavuk, M., Foushee, H. R., Carpenter, D. O., & Anniston Environmental Health Research Consortium (2011). "Blood pressure in relation to concentrations of PCB congeners and chlorinated pesticides." *Environmental Health Perspectives*, *119*(3), 319–325. https://doi.org/10.1289/ehp.1002830.

3  "Health implications of toxic chemical contamination of the Santa Monica Bay: hearing before the Subcommittee on Health and the Environment of the Committee on Energy and Commerce, House of Representatives, Ninety-ninth Congress,

second session, February 10, 1986." February 10, 1986. https://books.google.com /books?id=CcI22mIJuHIC&q= Retrieved April 26, 2023.

4   Gossett, R., Wikholm, G. Ljubenkov, J. & Steinman, D. (1989). "Human serum DDT levels related to consumption of fish from the coastal waters of Los Angeles," *Environmental Toxicology and Chemistry,* October. https://setac.onlinelibrary.wiley .com/doi/abs/10.1002/etc.5620081014.

5   Cone, M. "Chemical Firms Settle DDT Suit," *Los Angeles Times,* December 20, 2000. https://www.latimes.com/archives/la-xpm-2000-dec-20-me-2261-story.html.

6   Burger, J., Stern, A. H., & Gochfeld, M. (2005). "Mercury in commercial fish: optimizing individual choices to reduce risk." *Environmental health perspectives, 113*(3), 266–271. https://doi.org/10.1289/ehp.7315.

7   Jensen, I. J., Eilertsen, K. E., Otnæs, C., Mæhre, H. K., & Elvevoll, E. O. (2020). "An Update on the Content of Fatty Acids, Dioxins, PCBs and Heavy Metals in Farmed, Escaped and Wild Atlantic Salmon (*Salmo salar* L.) in Norway." *Foods (Basel, Switzerland), 9*(12), 1901. https://doi.org/10.3390/foods9121901.

8   Hodgson, Jessica. "Q&A: Salmon. As concern erupts over cancer-causing toxins in Scottish farmed salmon, Jessica Hodgson explains everything you need to know about the latest food scare." *The Guardian,* January 9, 2004. https://www.theguardian.com /environment/2004/jan/09/fishing.theissuesexplained.

9   Nicklisch, S., Bonito, L. T., Sandin, S., & Hamdoun, A. (2017). "Mercury levels of yellowfin tuna (Thunnus albacares) are associated with capture location." *Environmental Pollution (Barking, Essex: 1987), 229,* 87–93. https://doi.org/10.1016/j .envpol.2017.05.070.

10  Nicklisch, S. C. T., Bonito, L. T., Sandin, S., & Hamdoun, A. (2017). "Geographic Differences in Persistent Organic Pollutant Levels of Yellowfin Tuna." *Environmental Health Perspectives, 125*(6), 067014. https://doi.org/10.1289/EHP518.

11  Tarapore, P., & Ouyang, B. (2021). "Perfluoroalkyl Chemicals and Male Reproductive Health: Do PFOA and PFOS Increase Risk for Male Infertility?" *International Journal of Environmental Research and Public Health, 18*(7), 3794. https://doi.org/10.3390 /ijerph18073794.

12  Weintraub, M., & Birnbaum, L. S. (2008). "Catfish consumption as a contributor to elevated PCB levels in a non-Hispanic black subpopulation." *Environmental Research, 107*(3), 412–417. https://doi.org/10.1016/j.envres.2008.03.001.

13  "'Forever chemical' raises questions about carp pulled from Lake Winona, The invasive fish was removed to improve water quality and were intended for East Coast food markets," *Alexandria Echo Press,* November 24, 2021. https://www.echopress.com/ news/forever-chemical-raises-questions-about-carp-pulled-from-lake-winona.

14  Zeng, Y. H., Luo, X. J., Zheng, X. B., Tang, B., Wu, J. P., & Mai, B. X. (2014). "Species-specific bioaccumulation of halogenated organic pollutants and their metabolites in fish serum from an e-waste site, South China." *Archives of Environmental Contamination and Toxicology, 67*(3), 348–357. https://doi.org/10.1007/s00244-014-0040-8.

15 Brim, M. S., Alam, S. K., & Jenkins, L. G. (2001). "Organochlorine pesticides and heavy metals in muscle and ovaries of Gulf coast striped bass (Morone saxatilis) from the Apalachicola River, Florida, USA." *Journal of Environmental Science and Health. Part. B, Pesticides, Food Contaminants, and Agricultural Wastes, 36*(1), 15–27. https://doi.org/10.1081/pfc-100000913.

16 Feist, G. W., Webb, M. A., Gundersen, D. T., Foster, E. P., Schreck, C. B., Maule, A. G., & Fitzpatrick, M. S. (2005). "Evidence of detrimental effects of environmental contaminants on growth and reproductive physiology of white sturgeon in impounded areas of the Columbia River." *Environmental Health Perspectives, 113*(12), 1675–1682. https://doi.org/10.1289/ehp.8072.

17 Alavi, S. M. H., Barzegar-Fallah, S., Rahdar, P., Ahmadi, M. M., Yavari, M., Hatef, A., Golshan, M., & Linhart, O. (2021). "A Review on Environmental Contaminants-Related Fertility Threat in Male Fishes: Effects and Possible Mechanisms of Action Learned from Wildlife and Laboratory Studies." *Animals: An Open Access Journal from MDPI, 11*(10), 2817. https://doi.org/10.3390/ani11102817.

18 Wang, W., Batterman, S., Chernyak, S., & Nriagu, J. (2008). "Concentrations and risks of organic and metal contaminants in Eurasian caviar." *Ecotoxicology and Environmental Safety, 71*(1), 138–148. https://doi.org/10.1016/j.ecoenv.2007.06.007.

19 Guo, M., Zheng, G., Peng, J., Meng, D., Wu, H., Tan, Z., Li, F., & Zhai, Y. (2019). "Distribution of perfluorinated alkyl substances in marine shellfish along the Chinese Bohai Sea coast." *Journal of Environmental Science and Health. Part. B, Pesticides, Food Contaminants, and Agricultural Wastes, 54*(4), 271–280. https://doi.org/10.1080/036 01234.2018.1559570.

20 Hites, R. A., Foran, J. A., Carpenter, D. O., Hamilton, M. C., Knuth, B. A., & Schwager, S. J. (2004). "Global assessment of organic contaminants in farmed salmon." *Science (New York, N.Y.), 303*(5655), 226–229. https://doi.org/10.1126/science .1091447.

21 "Polychlorinated biphenyls (PCBs) in Alaska's Fish. Fish Samples collected: 2001–2021," Alaska Department of Environmental Conservation Office of the State Veterinarian Fish Monitoring Program file:///C:/Users/David/Downloads/pcb-in -alaska-fish-1.pdf.

22 Nathan, J. "Loathe gefilte fish? Not after you've tried this," *The New York Times*, April 12, 2016. https://www.nytimes.com/2016/04/13/dining/gefilte-fish-passover-recipes .html.

23 Skinner, L.C., Kane, M.W., Gottschall, K., & Simpson, D.A. "Chemical Residue Concentrations in Four Species of Fish and the American Lobster from Long Island Sound," Connecticut and New York: 2006 and 2007, New York State Department of Environmental Conservation Division of Fish, Wildlife and Marine Resources, 625 Broadway, Albany, NY 12233-4756; Connecticut Department of Environmental Protection Marine Resources Division, P. O. Box 719, Old Lyme,

CT, 06371. https://longislandsoundstudy.net/wp-content/uploads/2010/02/LISreport _110109FINALREPORT-1.pdf.

24  Young, W., Wiggins, S., Limm, W., Fisher, C. M., DeJager, L., & Genualdi, S. (2022). "Analysis of Per- and Poly(fluoroalkyl) Substances (PFASs) in Highly Consumed Seafood Products from U.S. Markets." *Journal of Agricultural and Food Chemistry*, *70*(42), 13545–13553. https://doi.org/10.1021/acs.jafc.2c04673.

25  Rodríguez-Hernández, Á., Camacho, M., Henríquez-Hernández, L. A., Boada, L. D., Valerón, P. F., Zaccaroni, A., Zumbado, M., Almeida-González, M., Rial-Berriel, C., & Luzardo, O. P. (2017). "Comparative study of the intake of toxic persistent and semi persistent pollutants through the consumption of fish and seafood from two modes of production (wild-caught and farmed)." *The Science of the Total Environment*, *575*, 919–931. https://doi.org/10.1016/j.scitotenv.2016.09.142.

26  de Boer, J., Lammertse, N., Koekkoek, J., & van Hattum, B. (2013). "PCB and organochlorine pesticide concentrations in eel increase after frying." *Chemosphere*, *90*(1), 139–142. https://doi.org/10.1016/j.chemosphere.2012.07.042.

27  Bayen, S., Barlow, P., Lee, H. K., & Obbard, J. P. (2005). "Effect of cooking on the loss of persistent organic pollutants from salmon." *Journal of Toxicology and Environmental Health. Part A*, *68*(4), 253–265. https://doi.org/10.1080/15287390590895126.

28  Storelli, M. M., Perrone, V. G., Busco, V. P., Spedicato, D., & Barone, G. (2012). "Persistent organic pollutants (PCBs and DDTs) in European conger eel, Conger con-ger L., from the Ionian Sea (Mediterranean Sea)." *Bulletin of environmental contami-nation and toxicology*, *88*(6), 928–932. https://doi.org/10.1007/s00128-012-0606-y.

29  "Advice for Pregnant Women on Fish Consumption concerning Mercury Contamination," Joint Sub-Committees on Animal Origin Foods and Toxicology under the Food Sanitation Committee the Pharmaceutical Affairs and Food Sanitation Council, June 3, 2003. https://www.mhlw.go.jp/english/wp/other/councils/mercury /index.html.

30  Nils-Gerrit Wunsch "Have you eaten any of the following raw foods in the past twelve months?" Statista.com, November 26, 2020. https://www.statista.com/statistics /947766/raw-food-meat-fish-consumption-us/.

31  Teas, J., Vena, S., Cone, D. L., & Irhimeh, M. (2013). "The consumption of seaweed as a protective factor in the etiology of breast cancer: proof of principle." *Journal of Applied Phycology*, *25*(3), 771–779. https://doi.org/10.1007/s10811-012-9931-0.

32  Maruyama, H., & Yamamoto, I. (1992). "Suppression of 125I-uptake in mouse thyroid by seaweed feeding: possible preventative effect of dietary seaweed on inter-nal radiation injury of the thyroid by radioactive iodine." *The Kitasato Archives of Experimental Medicine*, *65*(4), 209–216.

33  Hu, Y., Hu, F. B., & Manson, J. E. (2019). "Marine Omega-3 Supplementation and Cardiovascular Disease: An Updated Meta-Analysis of 13 Randomized Controlled Trials Involving 127 477 Participants." *Journal of the American Heart Association*, *8*(19), e013543. https://doi.org/10.1161/JAHA.119.013543.

34 de Boer, J., Lammertse, N., Koekkoek, J., & van Hattum, B. (2013). "PCB and organochlorine pesticide concentrations in eel increase after frying." *Chemosphere*, *90*(1), 139–142. https://doi.org/10.1016/j.chemosphere.2012.07.042.

35 HERO ID 2309353 Technical Report. "Residues of organochlorine pesticides in foods." Takamiya, T; Uchida, A 1978 Report Number PESTAB/79/0545 Jpn. J. Rural Med. https://hero.epa.gov/hero/index.cfm/reference/details/reference_id/2309353.

## Chapter 3

1 Jayaraj, R., Megha, P., & Sreedev, P. (2016). "Organochlorine pesticides, their toxic effects on living organisms and their fate in the environment." *Interdisciplinary Toxicology*, *9*(3-4), 90–100, https://doi.org/10.1515/intox-2016-0012.

2 Lean, I. J., Golder, H. M., Lees, N. M., McGilchrist, P., & Santos, J. E. P. (2018). "Effects of hormonal growth promotants on beef quality: a meta-analysis." *Journal of Animal Science*, *96*(7), 2675–2697. https://doi.org/10.1093/jas/sky123.

3 Jeong, S. H., Kang, D., Lim, M. W., Kang, C. S., & Sung, H. J. (2010). "Risk assessment of growth hormones and antimicrobial residues in meat." *Toxicological Research*, *26*(4), 301–313. https://doi.org/10.5487/TR.2010.26.4.301.

4 Jansen, E. C., Marín, C., Mora-Plazas, M., & Villamor, E. (2015). "Higher Childhood Red Meat Intake Frequency Is Associated with Earlier Age at Menarche." *The Journal of Nutrition*, *146*(4), 792–798, https://doi.org/10.3945/jn.115.226456.

5 Korenman S. G. (1980). "Oestrogen window hypothesis of the aetiology of breast cancer." *Lancet (London, England)*, *1*(8170), 700–701.

6 Afeiche, M. C., Williams, P. L., Gaskins, A. J., Mendiola, J., Jørgensen, N., Swan, S. H., & Chavarro, J. E. (2014). "Meat intake and reproductive parameters among young men." *Epidemiology (Cambridge, Mass.)*, *25*(3), 323–330. https://doi.org/10.1097/EDE.0000000000000092.

7 Swan, S. H., Liu, F., Overstreet, J. W., Brazil, C., & Skakkebaek, N. E. (2007). "Semen quality of fertile US males in relation to their mothers' beef consumption during pregnancy." *Human Reproduction (Oxford, England)*, *22*(6), 1497–1502. https://doi.org/10.1093/humrep/dem068.

8 Rignell-Hydbom, A., Lindh, C. H., Dillner, J., Jönsson, B. A., & Rylander, L. (2012). "A nested case-control study of intrauterine exposure to persistent organochlorine pollutants and the risk of hypospadias." *PloS one*, *7*(9), e44767. https://doi.org/10.1371/journal.pone.0044767.

9 Mason, S. E., Baynes, R. E., Buur, J. L., Riviere, J. E., & Almond, G. W. (2008). "Sulfamethazine water medication pharmacokinetics and contamination in a commercial pig production unit." *Journal of Food Protection*, *71*(3), 584–589. https://doi.org/10.4315/0362-028x-71.3.584.

10 Fan F. S. (2022). "Consumption of meat containing ractopamine might enhance tumor growth through induction of asparagine synthetase." *European Journal of*

*Cancer Prevention: The Official Journal of the European Cancer Prevention Organisation (ECP)*, *31*(1), 82–84. https://doi.org/10.1097/CEJ.0000000000000655.

11 Davis, H. E., Geornaras, I., Lindstrom, V., Chaparro, J. M., Nair, M. N., Delmore, R. J., Engle, T. E., Belk, K. E., & Prenni, J. E. (2020). "Effects of differing withdrawal times from ractopamine hydrochloride on residue concentrations of beef muscle, adipose tissue, rendered tallow, and large intestine." *PloS one*, *15*(12), e0242673. https://doi.org/10.1371/journal.pone.0242673.

12 Sun, L., Wang, S., Lin, X., Tan, H., & Fu, Z. (2016). "Early Life Exposure to Ractopamine Causes Endocrine-Disrupting Effects in Japanese Medaka (Oryzias latipes)." *Bulletin of Environmental Contamination and Toxicology*, *96*(2), 150–155. https://doi.org/10.1007/s00128-015-1659-5.

13 Segedie, L. "DDT testing of ButcherBox Organic Chicken & Ground Beef," Mamavation.com, November 4, 2020. https://www.mamavation.com/food/ddt-testing-butcherbox-organic-chicken-ground-beef.html.

14 Preston-Martin, S., Pogoda, J. M., Mueller, B. A., Holly, E. A., Lijinsky, W., & Davis, R. L. (1996). "Maternal consumption of cured meats and vitamins in relation to pediatric brain tumors." *Cancer Epidemiology, Biomarkers & Prevention : A Publication of the American Association for Cancer Research, Cosponsored by the American Society of Preventive Oncology*, *5*(8), 599–605.

15 Searles Nielsen, S., Mueller, B. A., Preston-Martin, S., Farin, F. M., Holly, E. A., & McKean-Cowdin, R. (2011). "Childhood brain tumors and maternal cured meat consumption in pregnancy: differential effect by glutathione S-transferases." *Cancer Epidemiology, Biomarkers & Prevention : A Publication of the American Association for Cancer Research, Cosponsored by the American Society of Preventive Oncology*, *20*(11), 2413–2419. https://doi.org/10.1158/1055-9965.EPI-11-0196.

16 Tannenbaum S. R. (1989). "Preventive action of vitamin C on nitrosamine formation. *International journal for vitamin and nutrition research.*" *Supplement Internationale Zeitschrift fur Vitamin- und Ernahrungsforschung*, supplement, 30, 109–113.

**Chapter 4**

1 Blayney, D.P. "The Changing Landscape of U.S. Milk Production," US Department of Agriculture, Electronic Report from the Economic Research Service, Statistical Bulletin 1978, June 2002. https://www.ers.usda.gov/webdocs/publications/47162/17864_sb978_1_.pdf.

2 MacDonald, J. M., Law, J., "Mosheim R. Consolidation in U.S. Dairy Farming," ERR-274, July 2020. https://www.ers.usda.gov/webdocs/publications/98901/err-274.pdf.

3 Sachi, S., Ferdous, J., Sikder, M. H., & Azizul Karim Hussani, S. M. (2019). "Antibiotic residues in milk: Past, present, and future." *Journal of Advanced Veterinary and Animal Research*, *6*(3), 315–332. https://doi.org/10.5455/javar.2019.f350.

4    Cornejo, J., Pokrant, E., Figueroa, F., Riquelme, R., Galdames, P., Di Pillo, F., Jimenez-Bluhm, P., & Hamilton-West, C. (2020). "Assessing Antibiotic Residues in Poultry Eggs from Backyard Production Systems in Chile, First Approach to a Non-Addressed Issue in Farm Animals." *Animals: An Open Access Journal from MDPI*, *10*(6), 1056. https://doi.org/10.3390/ani10061056.

5    Biello, D. "Monsanto puts bovine growth hormone out to pasture," *Scientific American*, August 7, 2008. https://blogs.scientificamerican.com/news-blog/monsanto -puts-bovine-growth-hormone-2008-08-07/.

6    Prosser, C. G., Fleet, I. R., & Corps, A. N. (1989). "Increased secretion of insulin-like growth factor I into milk of cows treated with recombinantly derived bovine growth hormone." *The Journal of Dairy Research*, *56*(1), 17–26. https://doi.org/10.1017 /s0022029900026170.

7    Epstein, S. S. (1996). "Unlabeled milk from cows treated with biosynthetic growth hormones: a case of regulatory abdication." *International Journal of Health Services: Planning, Administration, Evaluation*, *26*(1), 173–185. https://doi.org/10.2190 /EDK8-T5RC-LUMR-B2H7.

8    "What do 'cage-free' egg labels really mean?" Humane League, March 17, 2021. https://thehumaneleague.org/article/cage-free-eggs-means.

### Chapter 5

1    Garfield, L. "A startup for millennial parents is banking on a $55 billion food opportu- nity no one talks about," *Business Insider*, June 13, 2017. https://www.businessinsider .com/yumi-baby-food-delivery-2017-6.

2    "Gillibrand Pushes for Legislation to Limit Levels of Toxic Heavy Metals in Baby Food," Kirsten Gillibrand, US Senator for New York, April 19, 2022. https: //www.gillibrand.senate.gov/news/press/release/gillibrand-pushes-for-legislation -to-limit-levels-of-toxic-heavy-metals-in-baby-food/.

3    Rosenbloom, C. "Arsenic in rice: What is and isn't safe for adults and children," *The Washington Post*, October 15, 2021. https://www.washingtonpost.com/lifestyle /2021/10/15/rice-arsenic-risk-children-amount/.

4    National Toxicology Program (NTP, 1982). Carcinogenesis Bioassay of 2,6-Dicholoro- p-phenylenediamine (CAS No. 609-20-1) in F344 rats and B6C3F1 (Feed Study), Technical Report Series, TR 219, NTP, Research Triangle Park, NC.

5    US EPA, 2006. Memorandum. Report of the Cancer Assessment Review Committee PC Code 031301. Office of Prevention, Pesticides, and Toxic Substances, Washington DC.

6    US EPA, 1988. Memorandum, DCNA; Review of Ames Assay, Office of Pesticides and Toxic Substances, Tox Chem 311, Record No. 215047.

## Chapter 6

1   Rui, Y. & Xuan, T. J. "China Bans Pesticides Lindane and Endosulfan," CX Tech, March 15, 2019. https://www.caixinglobal.com/2019-03-15/china-bans-pesticides -lindane-and-endosulfan-101393255.html.

2   Jameson, H. R. (1958). "The mechanism of the control of turnip flea beetle by ben-zene hexachloride dressings on brassicae seed." *Journal of the Science of Food and Agriculture,* 9, 590-596.

3   Hearon, S. E., Wang, M., & Phillips, T. D. (2020). "Strong Adsorption of Dieldrin by Parent and Processed Montmorillonite Clays." *Environmental Toxicology and Chemistry, 39*(3), 517–525. https://doi.org/10.1002/etc.4642.

4   Meeker, J. D., Ryan, L., Barr, D. B., Herrick, R. F., Bennett, D. H., Bravo, R., & Hauser, R. (2004). "The relationship of urinary metabolites of carbaryl/naphtha-lene and chlorpyrifos with human semen quality." *Environmental Health Perspectives, 112*(17), 1665–1670. https://doi.org/10.1289/ehp.7234.

5   Kulshrestha, S. K., & Arora, N. (1984). "Impairments induced by sublethal doses of two pesticides in the ovaries of a freshwater teleost Channa striatus Bloch." *Toxicology Letters, 20*(1), 93–98. https://doi.org/10.1016/0378-4274(84)90189-9. PMID: 6420940.

6   Shelton, J. F., Geraghty, E. M., Tancredi, D. J., Delwiche, L. D., Schmidt, R. J., Ritz, B., Hansen, R. L., & Hertz-Picciotto, I. (2014). "Neurodevelopmental disorders and prenatal residential proximity to agricultural pesticides: the CHARGE study." *Environmental Health Perspectives, 122*(10), 1103–1109. https://doi.org/10.1289 /ehp.1307044.

## Chapter 7

1   Pilet, J. "Resilience in food safety for 2021: Consumer related challenges," *Food Safety News,* January 18, 2021. https://www.foodsafetynews.com/2021/01/resilience -in-food-safety-for-2021-consumer-related-challenges.

2   Cheryl D. Fryar, M.S.P.H, Margaret D. Carroll, M.S.P.H, Namanjeet Ahluwalia, Ph.D., and Cynthia L. Ogden, Ph.D. "Fast Food Intake Among Children and Adolescents in the United States," 2015–2018 NCHS Data Brief No. 375, August 2020. https://www.cdc.gov/nchs/products/databriefs/db375.htm.

3   Zota, A. R., Phillips, C. A., & Mitro, S. D. (2016). "Recent Fast Food Consumption and Bisphenol A and Phthalates Exposures among the U.S. Population in NHANES, 2003-2010." *Environmental Health Perspectives, 124*(10), 1521–1528. https://doi .org/10.1289/ehp.1510803.

4   Muncke, J., Andersson, A. M., Backhaus, T., Boucher, J. M., et al (2020). "Impacts of food contact chemicals on human health: a consensus statement." *Environmental Health: A Global Access Science Source, 19*(1), 25. https://doi.org/10.1186/s12940 -020-0572-5.

5   "Everything you ever wanted to know about how McDonald's food is made," *Business Insider India*, July 26, 2021. https://www.businessinsider.in/retail/everything-you-ever-wanted-to-know-about-how-mcdonalds-food-is-made/slidelist/47270850.cms#slideid=47270851.

6   "Where does Wendy's get their fresh beef from?" Wendys.com. https://www.wendys.com/blog/fresh-beef-you-ask-wendys-has-answer.

7   Hayes, A. "The Story Behind Shake Shack's Success," Investopedia.com, February 17, 2022. https://www.investopedia.com/articles/personal-finance/041615/story-behind-shake-shacks-success.asp.

8   "Frequently Asked Questions Where Does Your Beef Come From?" Burgerfi. https://www.burgerfi.com/faq/.

9   "Our Values," Chipotle.com. https://www.chipotle.com/values.

10  Lanhee Lee, J. "Burger King is testing a plant-based Impossible Whopper," *Reuters*, April 1, 2019. https://www.businessinsider.com/vegetarian-patty-gets-the-burger-king-whopper-test-2019-4.

11  Survey Data on Acrylamide in Food, Food and Drug Administration. https://www.fda.gov/food/process-contaminants-food/survey-data-acrylamide-food.

12  DePass, D. & Bjorhus, J. "3M idles part of its Alabama plant after PFAS chemicals found in Tennessee River and ground water," *Star Tribune*, September 20, 2019. https://www.startribune.com/3m-idles-part-of-its-alabama-plant-after-pfas-chemicals-found-in-tennesee-river-and-ground-water/560921532/.

13  Susmann, H. P., Schaider, L. A., Rodgers, K. M., & Rudel, R. A. (2019). "Dietary Habits Related to Food Packaging and Population Exposure to PFASs." *Environmental Health Perspectives*, 127(10), 107003. https://doi.org/10.1289/EHP4092.

14  Molloy, J. "New Report Reveals Scary Truth About Chemicals In Fast Food Packaging," Tastingtable.com, March 24, 2022. https://www.tastingtable.com/809975/new-report-reveals-scary-truth-about-chemicals-in-fast-food-packaging/.

15  Hirsh, S. "These Restaurants and Food Delivery Platforms Offer Reusable Takeout Containers," Green Matters, May 24, 2022. https://www.greenmatters.com/p/restaurants-reusable-returnable-containers.

16  "Number of Sweetgreen locations in the United States in 2023," Scrapeher, March 13, 2023. https://www.scrapehero.com/location-reports/Sweetgreen-USA/.

17  "We believe that food has the power to change the world," Chipotle.com https://www.chipotle.com/values.

18  "UPDATE - El Pollo Loco Improves Access to Better-For-You Food with New Pollo Fit Bowls Keto Friendly. Paleo Friendly. Life Friendly," Globe Newsire, December 27, 2019. https://investor.elpolloloco.com/news-releases/news-release-details/update-el-pollo-loco-improves-access-better-you-food-new-pollo.

19  "The Kid's Meal beverage is available at no extra cost," ChickFilA.com. https://www.chick-fil-a.com/stories/news/chick-fil-a-adds-first-organic-offering-to-menu.

20 "Panera Bread® Shares Animal Welfare Progress and Makes New Cage-Free Commitment," PaneraBread.com, November 5, 2015. https://www.panerabread.com/content/dam/panerabread/documents/press/2015/animal-welfare-press-release-11012015.pdf.

21 "Animal welfare policy," Subway. file:///C:/Users/David/Downloads/Subway-Animal-Welfare-Policy.pdf.

22 "Sustainable Packaging," Jack in the Box.com. https://investors.jackinthebox.com/esg/Sustainable-Packaging/.

23 "Jack in the Box using 'mostly' cage-free eggs," QSRWeb.com, October 1, 2020. https://www.qsrweb.com/news/jack-in-the-box-using-mostly-cage-free-eggs/.

24 Branch, J. "Most Fast-Food Chains Still Serve Beef Raised With Antibiotics," *Consumer Reports*, October 31, 2019. https://www.consumerreports.org/overuse-of-antibiotics/most-fast-food-chains-still-serve-beef-raised-with-antibiotics/.

25 "Wendy's is proud to serve fresh, never-frozen, North American fed-beef in restaurants in the contiguous U.S., Alaska and Canada," Wendys.com. https://www.wendys.com/csr-what-we-value/food/responsible-sourcing/beef.

26 "Wendy's announces ban on toxic chemicals in food packaging," Toxic-Free Future, April 28, 2021. https://toxicfreefuture.org/press-room/wendys-announces-ban-on-toxic-chemicals-in-food-packaging/.

27 "Nutrition & Allergen Information," FiveGuys.com. https://www.fiveguys.com/-/media/public-site/files/allergen-ingredients-and-nutrition-info/allergen-guide/nutrition-allergen-march-2018-us.ashx.

28 "Burger King announces global ban of toxic 'forever chemical' in food packaging," Toxic-Free Future, March 24, 2022.

29 Ibid.

30 Ibid.

31 Segedie, L. "Does In-N-Out Burger Contain Toxic PFAS? LAB REPORTS," Mammavation, September 15, 2020. https://www.mamavation.com/food/in-n-out-burger-pfas-lab-reports.html.

**Chapter 8**

1 Tomaszewska, E., Muszyński, S., Świetlicka, I., Wojtysiak, D., Dobrowolski, P., Arciszewski, M. B., Donaldson, J., Czech, A., Hułas-Stasiak, M., Kuc, D., & Mielnik-Błaszczak, M. (2022). "Prenatal acrylamide exposure results in time-dependent changes in liver function and basal hematological, and oxidative parameters in weaned Wistar rats." *Scientific Reports*, 12(1), 14882. https://doi.org/10.1038/s41598-022-19178-5.

2 Lam, S. K., To, W. K., Duthie, S. J., & Ma, H. K. (1992). "The effect of smoking during pregnancy on the incidence of low birth weight among Chinese parturients." *The Australian & New Zealand Journal of Obstetrics & Gynaecology*, 32(2), 125–128. https://doi.org/10.1111/j.1479-828x.1992.tb01923.x.

3 Timmermann, C., Mølck, S. S., Kadawathagedara, M., Bjerregaard, A. A., Törnqvist,

M., Brantsæter, A. L., & Pedersen, M. (2021). "A Review of Dietary Intake of Acrylamide in Humans." *Toxics, 9*(7), 155. https://doi.org/10.3390/toxics9070155.

4   Källén K. (2000). "Maternal smoking during pregnancy and infant head circumference at birth." *Early Human Development, 58*(3), 197–204. https://doi.org/10.1016/s0378-3782(00)00077-3.

5   Janneke G. Hogervorst, Leo J. Schouten, Erik J. Konings, R. Alexandra Goldbohm and Piet A. van den Brandt. (2007). "A Prospective Study of Dietary Acrylamide Intake and the Risk of Endometrial, Ovarian, and Breast Cancer," *Cancer Epidemiology Biomarkers & Prevention,* 16(11):2304–13DOI: 10.1158/1055-9965.EPI-07-0581.

6   Wilson, K. M., Mucci, L. A., Rosner, B. A., & Willett, W. C. (2010). "A prospective study on dietary acrylamide intake and the risk for breast, endometrial, and ovarian cancers." *Cancer Epidemiology, Biomarkers & Prevention: A Publication of the American Association for Cancer Research, Cosponsored by the American Society Of Preventive Oncology, 19*(10), 2503–2515. https://doi.org/10.1158/1055-9965.EPI-10-0391.

7   Bongers, M. L., Hogervorst, J. G., Schouten, L. J., Goldbohm, R. A., Schouten, H. C., & van den Brandt, P. A. (2012). "Dietary acrylamide intake and the risk of lymphatic malignancies: the Netherlands Cohort Study on diet and cancer." *PloS one, 7*(6), e38016. https://doi.org/10.1371/journal.pone.0038016.

8   Mead M. N. (2007). "Aspartame Cancer Risks Revisited: Prenatal Exposure May Be Greatest Concern." *Environmental Health Perspectives, 115*(9), A460.

9   Janneke G. Hogervorst, Leo J. Schouten, Erik J. Konings, R. Alexandra Goldbohm and Piet A. van den Brandt. (2007). "A Prospective Study of Dietary Acrylamide Intake and the Risk of Endometrial, Ovarian, and Breast Cancer," *Cancer Epidemiology Biomarkers & Prevention,* 16(11):2304–13DOI: 10.1158/1055-9965.EPI-07-0581.

10  Wilson, K. M., Mucci, L. A., Rosner, B. A., & Willett, W. C. (2010). "A prospective study on dietary acrylamide intake and the risk for breast, endometrial, and ovarian cancers." *Cancer Epidemiology, Biomarkers & Prevention: A Publication of the American Association for Cancer Research, Cosponsored by the American Society Of Preventive Oncology, 19*(10), 2503–2515. https://doi.org/10.1158/1055-9965.EPI-10-0391.

11  Bongers, M. L., Hogervorst, J. G., Schouten, L. J., Goldbohm, R. A., Schouten, H. C., & van den Brandt, P. A. (2012). "Dietary acrylamide intake and the risk of lymphatic malignancies: the Netherlands Cohort Study on dict and cancer." *PloS one, 7*(6), e38016. https://doi.org/10.1371/journal.pone.0038016.

12  Crawford, L. M., Kahlon, T. S., Chiu, M. M., Wang, S. C., & Friedman, M. (2019). "Acrylamide Content of Experimental and Commercial Flatbreads." *Journal of Food Science, 84*(3), 659–666. https://doi.org/10.1111/1750-3841.14456.

13  Curtis, T. Y., Postles, J., & Halford, N. G. (2014). "Reducing the potential for processing contaminant formation in cereal products." *Journal of Cereal Science, 59*(3), 382–392. https://doi.org/10.1016/j.jcs.2013.11.002.

14  R. M. Delgado, G. Ar ambula-Villa, G. Luna-B arcenas, V. Flores-Casamayor,

J.J. Veles-Medina, E. Azuara and R. Salazar. (2016) "Acrylamide Content in Tortilla Chips Prepared from Pigmented Maize Kernels." Revista Mexicana de Ingeniería Química, Vol. 15, No. 1 69-78. https://www.scielo.org.mx/pdf/rmiq/v15n1/1665-2738-rmiq-15-01-00069.pdf.

### Chapter 9

1  Hrubec, T. C., Seguin, R. P., Xu, L., Cortopassi, G. A., Datta, S., Hanlon, A. L., Lozano, A. J., McDonald, V. A., Healy, C. A., Anderson, T. C., Musse, N. A., & Williams, R. T. (2021). "Altered toxicological endpoints in humans from common quaternary ammonium compound disinfectant exposure." *Toxicology Reports*, 8, 646–656. https://doi.org/10.1016/j.toxrep.2021.03.006.

2  "Do You Know What's in Your Cosmetics?" *The New York Times*, February 9, 2019. https://www.nytimes.com/2019/02/09/opinion/cosmetics-safety-makeup.html

3  "50 beauty industry statistics to keep you on trend," Thimble.com, August 22, 2021. https://www.thimble.com/blog/beauty-industry-statistics.

4  "Beauty, Cosmetics & Fragrance Stores in the US - Employment Statistics 2003–2028, Ibisworld.com," August 30, 2022. https://www.ibisworld.com/industry-statistics/employment/beauty-cosmetics-fragrance-stores-united-states/.

5  "About the Cosmetic Ingredient Review," Cosmetic Ingredient Review. https://www.cir-safety.org/about.

6  "Amended Safety Assessment of Quaternium-18 and Quaternium-18 Bentonite as Used in Cosmetics Status: Draft Amended Rep," Cosmetic Ingredient Review, February 21, 2020. https://www.cir-safety.org/sites/default/files/Quaternium-18_0.pdf.

7  Melin, V. E., Potineni, H., Hunt, P., Griswold, J., Siems, B., Werre, S. R., & Hrubec, T. C. (2014). "Exposure to common quaternary ammonium disinfectants decreases fertility in mice." *Reproductive Toxicology (Elmsford, N.Y.)*, 50, 163–170. https://doi.org/10.1016/j.reprotox.2014.07.071.

8  Melin, V. E., Melin, T. E., Dessify, B. J., Nguyen, C. T., Shea, C. S., & Hrubec, T. C. (2016). "Quaternary ammonium disinfectants cause subfertility in mice by targeting both male and female reproductive processes." *Reproductive Toxicology (Elmsford, N.Y.)*, 59, 159–166. https://doi.org/10.1016/j.reprotox.2015.10.006.

9  Hrubec, T. C., Melin, V. E., Shea, C. S., Ferguson, E. E., Garofola, C., Repine, C. M., Chapman, T. W., Patel, H. R., Razvi, R. M., Sugrue, J. E., Potineni, H., Magnin-Bissel, G., & Hunt, P. A. (2017). "Ambient and Dosed Exposure to Quaternary Ammonium Disinfectants Causes Neural Tube Defects in Rodents." *Birth Defects Research*, 109(14), 1166–1178. https://doi.org/10.1002/bdr2.1064.

10  Hrubec, T. C., Seguin, R. P., Xu, L., Cortopassi, G. A., Datta, S., Hanlon, A. L., Lozano, A. J., McDonald, V. A., Healy, C. A., Anderson, T. C., Musse, N. A., & Williams, R. T. (2021). "Altered toxicological endpoints in humans from common

quaternary ammonium compound disinfectant exposure." *Toxicology Reports, 8,* **646**–656. https://doi.org/10.1016/j.toxrep.2021.03.006.

11  COMMISSION REGULATION (EU) 2019/831 of 22 May 2019 amending Annexes II, III and V to Regulation (EC) No 1223/2009 of the European Parliament and of the Council on cosmetic products, Official Journal of the European Union. https://eur-lex.europa.eu/legal-content/EN/TXT/PDF/?uri=CELEX:32019R0831&rid=1.

12  "Are Quats/QACs allowed in EU?" International Food Safety & Quality Network, September 28, 2018. htps://www.ifsqn.com/forum/index.php/topic/33268-are-quatsqacs-allowed-in-eu/.

13  "Cosmetics Committee Approves Three Cosmetic Ingredients," UL Solutions, November 11, 2015. https://www.ul.com/news/cosmetics-committee-approves-three-cosmetic-ingredients.

14  Zota, A. R., & Shamasunder, B. (2017). "The environmental injustice of beauty: framing chemical exposures from beauty products as a health disparities concern." *American Journal of Obstetrics and Gynecology, 217*(4), 418.e1–418.e6. https://doi.org/10.1016/j.ajog.2017.07.020.

15  Eltoukhi, H. M., Modi, M. N., Weston, M., Armstrong, A. Y., & Stewart, E. A. (2014). "The health disparities of uterine fibroid tumors for African American women: a public health issue." *American Journal of Obstetrics and Gynecology, 210*(3), 194–199. https://doi.org/10.1016/j.ajog.2013.08.008.

16  Ellington T. D., Henley S. J., Wilson R. J., Miller J. W., Wu M., Richardson L. C. (2022). "Trends in breast cancer mortality by race/ethnicity, age, and US Census Region, United States—1999–2020," *Cancer,* 129(1), pp. 32–38. doi:10.1002/cncr.34503.

17  Eberle, C. E., Sandler, D. P., Taylor, K. W., & White, A. J. (2020). "Hair dye and chemical straightener use and breast cancer risk in a large US population of black and white women." *International Journal of Cancer, 147*(2), 383–391. https://doi.org/10.1002/ijc.32738.

18  Helm, J. S., Nishioka, M., Brody, J. G., Rudel, R. A., & Dodson, R. E. (2019). "Re: Measurement of endocrine disrupting and asthma-associated chemicals in hair products used by Black women." *Environmental Research, 172,* 719–721. https://doi.org/10.1016/j.envres.2018.11.029.

19  Byford, J. R., Shaw, L. E., Drew, M. G., Pope, G. S., Sauer, M. J., & Darbre, P. D. (2002). "Oestrogenic activity of parabens in MCF7 human breast cancer cells." *The Journal of Steroid Biochemistry and Molecular Biology, 80*(1), 49–60. https://doi.org/10.1016/s0960-0760(01)00174-1.

20  Darbre, P. D., Aljarrah, A., Miller, W. R., Coldham, N. G., Sauer, M. J., & Pope, G. S. (2004). "Concentrations of parabens in human breast tumours." *Journal of Applied Toxicology: JAT, 24*(1), 5–13. https://doi.org/10.1002/jat.958.

21  Chemical Toxin Working Group, English Leather Cologne Splash 8.0 fl. oz (236 ml), Ellipse Analytics, March 4, 2021 Lot #: 19323A.

22  Chemical Toxin Working Group, Navy for Women Cologne Spray 1.5 fl. Oz (45 ml), Ellipse Analytics, March 4, 2021 Lot #: 19245A.

23  Park, S., Kim, B. N., Cho, S. C., Kim, Y., Kim, J. W., Lee, J. Y., Hong, S. B., Shin, M. S., Yoo, H. J., Im, H., Cheong, J. H., & Han, D. H. (2014). "Association between urine phthalate levels and poor attentional performance in children with attention-deficit hyperactivity disorder with evidence of dopamine gene-phthalate interaction." *International Journal of Environmental Research and Public Health*, *11*(7), 6743–6756. https://doi.org/10.3390/ijerph110706743.

24  Park, S., Lee, J. M., Kim, J. W., Cheong, J. H., Yun, H. J., Hong, Y. C., Kim, Y., Han, D. H., Yoo, H. J., Shin, M. S., Cho, S. C., & Kim, B. N. (2015). "Association between phthalates and externalizing behaviors and cortical thickness in children with attention deficit hyperactivity disorder." *Psychological Medicine*, *45*(8), 1601–1612. https://doi.org/10.1017/S0033291714002694.

25  Park, S., Kim, B. N., Cho, S. C., Kim, Y., Kim, J. W., Lee, J. Y., Hong, S. B., Shin, M. S., Yoo, H. J., Im, H., Cheong, J. H., & Han, D. H. (2014). "Association between urine phthalate levels and poor attentional performance in children with attention-deficit hyperactivity disorder with evidence of dopamine gene-phthalate interaction." *International Journal of Environmental Research and Public Health*, *11*(7), 6743–6756. https://doi.org/10.3390/ijerph110706743.

26  Percy, Z., Xu, Y., Sucharew, H., Khoury, J. C., Calafat, A. M., Braun, J. M., Lanphear, B. P., Chen, A., & Yolton, K. (2016). "Gestational exposure to phthalates and gender-related play behaviors in 8-year-old children: an observational study." *Environmental Health: A Global Access Science Source*, *15*(1), 87. https://doi.org/10.1186/s12940-016-0171-7.

27  Evans, S. F., Raymond, S., Sethuram, S., Barrett, E. S., Bush, N. R., Nguyen, R., Sathyanarayana, S., & Swan, S. H. (2021). "Associations between prenatal phthalate exposure and sex-typed play behavior in preschool age boys and girls." *Environmental Research*, *192*, 110264. https://doi.org/10.1016/j.envres.2020.110264.

28  Hlisníková, H., Petrovičová, I., Kolena, B., Šidlovská, M., & Sirotkin, A. (2020). "Effects and Mechanisms of Phthalates' Action on Reproductive Processes and Reproductive Health: A Literature Review." *International Journal of Environmental Research and Public Health*, *17*(18), 6811. https://doi.org/10.3390/ijerph17186811.

29  Basso, C. G., de Araújo-Ramos, A. T., & Martino-Andrade, A. J. (2022). "Exposure to phthalates and female reproductive health: A literature review." *Reproductive Toxicology (Elmsford, N.Y.)*, *109*, 61–79. https://doi.org/10.1016/j.reprotox.2022.02.006.

30  Park, S., Kim, B. N., Cho, S. C., Kim, Y., Kim, J. W., Lee, J. Y., Hong, S. B., Shin, M. S., Yoo, H. J., Im, H., Cheong, J. H., & Han, D. H. (2014). "Association between urine phthalate levels and poor attentional performance in children with attention-deficit hyperactivity disorder with evidence of dopamine gene-phthalate

interaction." *International Journal of Environmental Research and Public Health*, *11*(7), 6743–6756. https://doi.org/10.3390/ijerph110706743.

31 Park, S., Lee, J. M., Kim, J. W., Cheong, J. H., Yun, H. J., Hong, Y. C., Kim, Y., Han, D. H., Yoo, H. J., Shin, M. S., Cho, S. C., & Kim, B. N. (2015). "Association between phthalates and externalizing behaviors and cortical thickness in children with attention deficit hyperactivity disorder." *Psychological Medicine*, *45*(8), 1601–1612. https://doi.org/10.1017/S0033291714002694.

32 Rowdhwal, S. S. S., & Chen, J. (2018). "Toxic Effects of Di-2-ethylhexyl Phthalate: An Overview." *BioMed Research International*, *2018*, 1750368. https://doi.org /10.1155/2018/1750368.

33 "U.S. population: Which brands of body and baby powder do you use most often?" Statista Research Department, June 23, 2022. https://www.statista.com/ statistics/275421/us-households-brands-of-body-and-bab-y-powder-used/.

34 "Johnson & Johnson's share of the baby care market worldwide from 2013 to 2021," Statista Research Department, Jul 17, 2014. https://www.statista.com /statistics/258429/johnson-und-johnsons-share-of-the-baby-care-market-worldwide/.

35 Lucaccioni, L., Trevisani, V., Passini, E., Righi, B., Plessi, C., Predieri, B., & Iughetti, L. (2021). "Perinatal Exposure to Phthalates: From Endocrine to Neurodevelopment Effects." *International Journal of Molecular Sciences*, *22*(8), 4063. https://doi.org /10.3390/ijms22084063.

36 Harley, K. G., Kogut, K., Madrigal, D. S., Cardenas, M., Vera, I. A., Meza-Alfaro, G., She, J., Gavin, Q., Zahedi, R., Bradman, A., Eskenazi, B., & Parra, K. L. (2016). "Reducing Phthalate, Paraben, and Phenol Exposure from Personal Care Products in Adolescent Girls: Findings from the HERMOSA Intervention Study." *Environmental Health Perspectives*, *124*(10), 1600–1607. https://doi.org/10.1289/ehp.1510514.

37 Stoker, T. E., Gibson, E. K., & Zorrilla, L. M. (2010). "Triclosan exposure modulates estrogen-dependent responses in the female wistar rat." *Toxicological Sciences: An Official Journal of the Society of Toxicology*, *117*(1), 45–53. https://doi.org/10.1093 /toxsci/kfq180.

38 1,4-DIOXANE (Group 2B), International Agency for Research on Cancer (IARC), 1991; 71:589 https://www.inchem.org/documents/iarc/vol71/019-dioxane.html.

39 "P&G reformulating to reduce 1,4-dioxane?" *HBW Insight*, March 22, 2010. https: //hbw.pharmaintelligence.informa.com/.

40 David Steinman v. The Procter and Gamble Distributing LLC Consent Judgement, Superior Court of the State of California County of San Francisco, Case No. CGC-10-500758, July 30, 2010. https://oag.ca.gov/system/files/prop65/judgments /2010-00119J1103.pdf.

41 "Healthy Nail Salons," California Healthy Nail Salon Collaborative. https://www .cahealthynailsalons.org/healthy-nail-salon.

42 Marques, A. C., Mariana, M., & Cairrao, E. (2022). "Triclosan and Its Consequences

on the Reproductive, Cardiovascular and Thyroid Levels." *International Journal of Molecular Sciences, 23*(19), 11427. https://doi.org/10.3390/ijms231911427.

43 "DevaCurl Maker Hit with Lawsuits Over Hair Loss, Scalp Irritation," Classaction.org January 10, 2022. https://www.classaction.org/devacurl-hair-loss-scalp-irritation-lawsuits.

44 Taylor, N. E., Kolton, E. A. "New Cosmetic Regulatory Requirements: What Cosmetic Manufacturers Need to Know," GreenbergTraurig, December 30, 2022. https://www.gtlaw.com/en/insights/2022/12/new-cosmetic-regulatory-requirements-what-cosmetic-manufacturers-need-to-know.

45 This legislation was included in H.R. 2617, the Consolidated Appropriations Act, 2023, as part of a year-end bill.

## Chapter 10

1 Sorg, L. "Susan Wind had a reason to press state officials about a possible cancer cluster near Lake Norman. Her daughter had the disease." *NC Policy Watch*, June 21, 2018. https://ncpolicywatch.com/2018/06/21/susan-wind-had-a-reason-to-press-state-officials-about-a-possible-cancer-cluster-near-lake-norman-her-daughter-had-the-disease/.

2 Beach, M. "Coal Ash Uncovered Near Lake Norman High School in Mooresville," WCCB Charlotte, October 24, 2018. https://www.wccbcharlotte.com/2018/10/24/coal-ash-uncovered-near-lake-norman-high-school-in-mooresville/.

3 Suggs, M. "Mooresville's 'Coal Ash Corridor' is largest concentration in state," *Mooresville Tribune*, October 27, 2018. https://mooresvilletribune.com/news/local/mooresvilles-coal-ash-corridor-is-largest-concentration-in-state/article_decd08c2-da1e-11e8-96f2-f7d911d2c512.html.

4 "Accidents at Nuclear Power Plants and Cancer Risk," National Cancer Institute. https://www.cancer.gov/about-cancer/causes-prevention/risk/radiation/nuclear-accidents-fact-sheet.

5 Fiore, M., Oliveri Conti, G., Caltabiano, R., Buffone, A., Zuccarello, P., Cormaci, L., Cannizzaro, M. A., & Ferrante, M. (2019). "Role of Emerging Environmental Risk Factors in Thyroid Cancer: A Brief Review." *International Journal of Environmental Research and Public Health, 16*(7), 1185. https://doi.org/10.3390/ijerph16071185.

6 Hu, M. J., He, J. L., Tong, X. R., Yang, W. J., Zhao, H. H., Li, G. A., & Huang, F. (2021). "Associations between essential microelements exposure and the aggressive clinicopathologic characteristics of papillary thyroid cancer." *Biometals: An International Journal on the Role of Metal Ions in Biology, Biochemistry, and Medicine, 34*(4), 909–921. https://doi.org/10.1007/s10534-021-00317-w.

7 "Manganese Occurrence Near Three Coal Ash Impoundments in Illinois," Electric Power Research Institute, September 24, 2002. https://www.epri.com/research/products/1005257.

8   "Nuclear Power Plants in Europe," European Nuclear Society, March 2022. https://www.euronuclear.org/glossary/nuclear-power-plants-in-europe/.

9   "List of Power Reactor Units," US Nuclear Regulatory Commission, December 30, 2022. https://www.nrc.gov/reactors/operating/list-power-reactor-units.html.

10  Power Plants and Neighboring Communities. https://www.epa.gov/airmarkets/power -plants-and-neighboring-communities.

11  Harvey, F. "Too many new coal-fired plants planned for 1.5C climate goal, report concludes," *The Guardian*, April 26, 2022. https://www.theguardian.com/environment /2022/apr/26/too-many-new-coal-fired-plants-planned-for-15c-climate-goal-report -concludes.

12  Lydersen, K. "Analysis finds 'stunning' lack of compliance with coal ash rules, putting groundwater at risk," Energy News Network, November 3, 2022. https://energynews .us/2022/11/03/analysis-finds-stunning-lack-of-compliance-with-coal-ash-rules -putting-groundwater-at-risk/.

13  "2017 Update on U.S. Oil & Gas Activity," Fractracker Alliance. https://www .fractracker.org/map/national/us-oil-gas/.

14  Tabuchi, H. "E.P.A. Approved Toxic Chemicals for Fracking a Decade Ago, New Files Show," *The New York Times*, July 12, 2021. https://www.nytimes.com/2021/07/12 /climate/epa-pfas-fracking-forever-chemicals.html.

15  Glassmeyer, S. T., Furlong, E. T., Kolpin, D. W., Batt, A. L., Benson, R., Boone, J. S., Conerly, O., Donohue, M. J., King, D. N., Kostich, M. S., Mash, H. E., Pfaller, S. L., Schenck, K. M., Simmons, J. E., Varughese, E. A., Vesper, S. J., Villegas, E. N., & Wilson, V. S. (2017). "Nationwide reconnaissance of contaminants of emerging concern in source and treated drinking waters of the United States." *The Science of the Total Environment*, *581-582*, 909–922. https://doi.org/10.1016/j.scitotenv.2016.12.004.

16  Hayes, J. "Most of DOD sites with 'forever chemicals' contamination exceed EPA health levels," Environmental Working Group, July 12, 2022.

17  "Mapping the PFAS contamination crisis: New data show 2,854 sites in 50 states and two territories," Environmental Working Group. https://www.ewg.org/interactive -maps/pfas_contamination/.

18  Shrestha, P. M., Humphrey, J. L., Carlton, E. J., Adgate, J. L., Barton, K. E., Root, E. D., & Miller, S. L. (2019). "Impact of Outdoor Air Pollution on Indoor Air Quality in Low-Income Homes during Wildfire Seasons." *International Journal of Environmental Research and Public Health*, *16*(19), 3535. https://doi.org/10.3390/ijerph16193535.

19  Perera, F. P., Li, Z., Whyatt, R., Hoepner, L., Wang, S., Camann, D., & Rauh, V. (2009). "Prenatal airborne polycyclic aromatic hydrocarbon exposure and child IQ at age 5 years." *Pediatrics*, *124*(2), e195–e202. https://doi.org/10.1542/peds.2008-3506.

20  Ulziikhuu, B., Gombojav, E., Banzrai, C., Batsukh, S., Enkhtuya, E., Boldbaatar, B., Bellinger, D. C., Lanphear, B. P., McCandless, L. C., Tamana, S. K., & Allen, R. W. (2022). "Portable HEPA Filter Air Cleaner Use during Pregnancy and Children's

Cognitive Performance at Four Years of Age: The UGAAR Randomized Controlled Trial." *Environmental Health Perspectives, 130*(6), 67006. https://doi.org/10.1289/EHP10302.

21 Dubey, S., Rohra, H., & Taneja, A. (2021). "Assessing effectiveness of air purifiers (HEPA) for controlling indoor particulate pollution." *Heliyon, 7*(9), e07976. https://doi.org/10.1016/j.heliyon.2021.e07976.

22 Claudio L. (2011). "Planting healthier indoor air." *Environmental Health Perspectives, 119*(10), A426–A427. https://doi.org/10.1289/ehp.119-a426.

23 Teiri, H., Pourzamzni, H., & Hajizadeh, Y. (2018). "Phytoremediation of Formaldehyde from Indoor Environment by Ornamental Plants: An Approach to Promote Occupants Health." *International Journal of Preventive Medicine, 9*, 70. https://doi.org/10.4103/ijpvm.IJPVM_269_16.

24 King, Anthony. "Trees Tested as Pollutant Traps. Silver birch, elder, and yew win out in an experiment to see which species best capture the tiny particles from diesel pollution," *The Scientist*, May 28, 2019. https://www.the-scientist.com/news-opinion/trees-tested-as-pollutant-traps-65940.

25 Kim, D., & Ahn, Y. (2021). "The Contribution of Neighborhood Tree and Greenspace to Asthma Emergency Room Visits: An Application of Advanced Spatial Data in Los Angeles County." *International Journal of Environmental Research and Public Health, 18*(7), 3487. https://doi.org/10.3390/ijerph18073487.

26 Isaifan, R. J., & Baldauf, R. W. (2020). "Estimating economic and environmental benefits of urban trees in desert regions." *Urban Forestry & Urban Greening, N/A*, 10.3389/fevo.2020.00016. https://doi.org/10.3389/fevo.2020.00016.

27 Nguyen, H. "Most Americans take their shoes off at home, but don't expect their guests to," Yougov.com, January 18, 2018. https://today.yougov.com/topics/society/articles-reports/2018/01/17/most-americans-take-their-shoes-home-dont-expect-t.

28 Harley, K. G., Parra, K. L., Camacho, J., Bradman, A., Nolan, J., Lessard, C., Anderson, K. A., Poutasse, C. M., Scott, R. P., Lazaro, G., Cardoso, E., Gallardo, D., & Gunier, R. B. (2019). "Determinants of pesticide concentrations in silicone wristbands worn by Latina adolescent girls in a California farmworker community: The COSECHA youth participatory action study." *The Science of the Total Environment, 652*, 1022–1029. https://doi.org/10.1016/j.scitotenv.2018.10.276.

29 Leppänen, M., Peräniemi, S., Koponen, H., Sippula, O., & Pasanen, P. (2020). "The effect of the shoeless course on particle concentrations and dust composition in schools." *The Science of the Total Environment, 710*, 136272. https://doi.org/10.1016/j.scitotenv.2019.136272.

30 Wiwanitkit V. (2011). "Nuclear detonation, thyroid cancer and potassium iodide prophylaxis." *Indian Journal of Endocrinology and Metabolism, 15*(2), 96–98. https://doi.org/10.4103/2230-8210.81937.

31 Genuis, S. J., Curtis, L., & Birkholz, D. (2013). "Gastrointestinal Elimination of

Perfluorinated Compounds Using Cholestyramine and Chlorella pyrenoidosa." *ISRN Toxicology*, *2013*, 657849. https://doi.org/10.1155/2013/657849.

32  Morita, K., Matsueda, T., Iida, T., & Hasegawa, T. (1999). "Chlorella accelerates dioxin excretion in rats." *The Journal of Nutrition*, *129*(9), 1731–1736. https://doi.org/10.1093/jn/129.9.1731.

33  Friedman, L. "In 'Cancer Alley,' Judge Blocks Huge Petrochemical Plant," *The New York Times*, September 15, 2022. https://www.nytimes.com/2022/09/15/climate/louisiana-judge-blocks-formosa-plant.html.

34  Villela Filho, M., Araujo, C., Bonfá, A., & Porto, W. (2011). "Chemistry based on renewable raw materials: perspectives for a sugar cane-based biorefinery." *Enzyme Research*, *2011*, 654596. https://doi.org/10.4061/2011/654596.

35  "Braskem's bioplastic recognized as one of Brazil's most transformational cases in sustainable development," Bioplasticsmagazine.com, June 2, 2020. https://www.bioplasticsmagazine.com/en/news/meldungen/20200601Braskem-s-bioplastic-recognized-as-one-of-Brazil-s-most-transformational-cases-in-sustainable-development.php.

## Chapter 11

1  Frisch, T. "Contamination Crisis, But Not an Official Response," *In These Times*, September 5, 2017. https://inthesetimes.com/article/industrial-pollution-pfoa-drinking-water-contamination-epa-saint-gobain.

2  Lyons, B. J. "A danger that lurks below. In Hoosick Falls, have health problems resulted from water contamination?" *Times Union*, Dec. 12, 2015. https://www.timesunion.com/local/article/A-danger-that-lurks-below-6694498.php.

3  Lyons, B. J. "A man's crusade culminated with massive PFOA settlements," *Times Union*, December 27, 2021. https://www.timesunion.com/state/article/A-man-s-crusade-culminated-with-massive-PFOA-16726257.php.

4  Waller, K., Swan, S. H., DeLorenze, G., & Hopkins, B. (1998). "Trihalomethanes in drinking water and spontaneous abortion." *Epidemiology (Cambridge, Mass.)*, *9*(2), 134–140.

5  Brown, K. W., Gessesse, B., Butler, L. J., & MacIntosh, D. L. (2017). "Potential Effectiveness of Point-of-Use Filtration to Address Risks to Drinking Water in the United States." *Environmental Health Insights*, *11*, 1178630217746997. https://doi.org/10.1177/1178630217746997.

6  Herkert, N. et al., "Assessing the Effectiveness of Point-of-Use Residential Drinking Water Filters for Perfluoroalkyl Substances (PFAS)," *Environmental Science & Technology* Letters 2020 7 (3), 178-184 DOI: 10.1021/acs.estlett.0c00004.

7  Patterson, C., Burkhardt, J., Schupp, D., Krishnan, E. R., Dyment, S., Merritt, S., Zintek, L., & Kleinmaier, D. (2019). "Effectiveness of point-of-use/point-of-entry

systems to remove per- and polyfluoroalkyl substances from drinking water." *AWWA Water Science*, *1*(2), 1–12. https://doi.org/10.1002/aws2.1131.

8 Patterson, C., Burkhardt, J., Schupp, D., Krishnan, E. R., Dyment, S., Merritt, S., Zintek, L., & Kleinmaier, D. (2019). "Effectiveness of point-of-use/point-of-entry systems to remove per- and polyfluoroalkyl substances from drinking water." *AWWA Water Science*, *1*(2), 1–12. https://doi.org/10.1002/aws2.1131.

9 "Removing Toxic Fluorinated Chemicals From Your Home's Tap Water," Environmental Working Group, March 10, 2021. https://www.ewg.org/news-insights /news/2018/09/removing-toxic-fluorinated-chemicals-your-homes-tap-water.

10 Brown, K. W., Gessesse, B., Butler, L. J., & MacIntosh, D. L. (2017). "Potential Effectiveness of Point-of-Use Filtration to Address Risks to Drinking Water in the United States." *Environmental Health Insights, 11*, 1178630217746997. https://doi .org/10.1177/1178630217746997.

11 Brown, K. W., Gessesse, B., Butler, L. J., & MacIntosh, D. L. (2017). "Potential Effectiveness of Point-of-Use Filtration to Address Risks to Drinking Water in the United States." *Environmental Health Insights, 11*, 1178630217746997. https://doi .org/10.1177/1178630217746997.

12 Boch, R. "Can Distillation Remove PFAS From Water? What the Experts Say," Purewaterblog.com. https://purewaterblog.com/can-distillation-remove-pfas-from -water-what-the-experts-say.

13 National Research Council (US) Committee on Contaminated Drinking Water at Camp Lejeune. Contaminated Water Supplies at Camp Lejeune: Assessing Potential Health Effects. Washington (DC): National Academies Press (US); 2009. 3, Systemic Exposures to Volatile Organic Compounds and Factors Influencing Susceptibility to Their Effects. Available from: https://www.ncbi.nlm.nih.gov/books/NBK215288/.

## Chapter 12

1 Harley, K. G., Calderon, L., Nolan, J., Maddalena, R., Russell, M., Roman, K., Mayo-Burgos, S., Cabrera, J., Morga, N., & Bradman, A. (2021). "Changes in Latina Women's Exposure to Cleaning Chemicals Associated with Switching from Conventional to 'Green' Household Cleaning Products: The LUCIR Intervention Study." *Environmental Health Perspectives*, *129*(9), 97001. https://doi.org/10.1289 /EHP8831.

2 Ibid.

3 Ibid.

4 Cordier, S, R Garlantézec, L Labat, F Rouget, C Monfort, N Bonvallot, B Roig, J Pulkkinen, C Chevrier and L Multigner. 2012. "Exposure during pregnancy to glycol ethers and chlorinated solvents and the risk of congenital malformations." *Epidemiology.* http://dx.doi.org/10.1097/EDE.0b013e31826c2bd8; Fabian Melchior Gerster, David Vernez, Pascal Pierre Wild, and Nancy Brenna Hopf. "Hazardous

substances in frequently used professional cleaning products," *Int J Occup Environ Health*. 2014 Mar; 20(1): 46–60. doi: 10.1179/2049396713Y.0000000052.

5  Liu X, Lao XQ, Wong CC, Tan L, Zhang Z, Wong TW, Tse LA, Lau AP, Yu IT. "Frequent use of household cleaning products is associated with rhinitis in Chinese children." *J Allergy Clin Immunol*. 2016. Sep;138(3):754-760.e6. doi: 10.1016/j .jaci.2016.03.038. Epub 2016 May 6.

6  Fabian MelchZahm, S. H., & Ward, M. H. (1998). "Pesticides and childhood cancer." *Environmental Health Perspectives, 106 Suppl 3*(Suppl 3), 893–908. https://doi .org/10.1289/ehp.98106893.

7  Gerster, F. M., Vernez, D., Wild, P. P., & Hopf, N. B. (2014). "Hazardous substances in frequently used professional cleaning products." *International Journal of Occupational and Environmental Health, 20*(1), 46–60. https://doi.org/10.1179/2049 396713Y.0000000052.

8  Mitro, S. D., Dodson, R. E., Singla, V., Adamkiewicz, G., Elmi, A. F., Tilly, M. K., & Zota, A. R. (2016). "Consumer Product Chemicals in Indoor Dust: A Quantitative Meta-analysis of U.S. Studies." *Environmental Science & Technology, 50*(19), 10661–10672. https://doi.org/10.1021/acs.est.6b02023.

9  Yu, C. H., Yiin, L. M., Tina Fan, Z. H., & Rhoads, G. G. (2009). "Evaluation of HEPA vacuum cleaning and dry steam cleaning in reducing levels of polycyclic aromatic hydrocarbons and house dust mite allergens in carpets." *Journal of Environmental Monitoring: JEM, 11*(1), 205–211. https://doi.org/10.1039/b807821a.

10  Harley, K. G., Parra, K. L., Camacho, J., Bradman, A., Nolan, J., Lessard, C., Anderson, K. A., Poutasse, C. M., Scott, R. P., Lazaro, G., Cardoso, E., Gallardo, D., & Gunier, R. B. (2019). "Determinants of pesticide concentrations in silicone wristbands worn by Latina adolescent girls in a California farmworker community: The COSECHA youth participatory action study." *The Science of the Total Environment, 652*, 1022–1029. https://doi.org/10.1016/j.scitotenv.2018.10.276.

11  Yiin, L. M., Rhoads, G. G., Rich, D. Q., Zhang, J., Bai, Z., Adgate, J. L., Ashley, P. J., & Lioy, P. J. (2002). "Comparison of techniques to reduce residential lead dust on carpet and upholstery: the new jersey assessment of cleaning techniques trial." *Environmental Health Perspectives, 110*(12), 1233–1237. https://doi.org/10.1289/ehp .021101233.

12  Persellin, K. "Toxic PFAS Chemicals Found in Period-Proof Underwear," February 21, 2020. https://pfasproject.com/2020/02/21/toxic-pfas-chemicals-found-in-period -proof-underwear/.

13  "Flame Retardants in Furniture. Furniture flame retardants harm our health and do not prevent fires," Green Science Policy Institute. https://greensciencepolicy.org /our-work/furniture/.

14  Ceballos, D. M., Fellows, K. M., Evans, A. E., Janulewicz, P. A., Lee, E. G., & Whittaker, S. G. (2021). "Perchloroethylene and Dry Cleaning: It's Time to Move

the Industry to Safer Alternatives." *Frontiers in Public Health*, *9*, 638082. https://doi
.org/10.3389/fpubh.2021.638082.

15 Yiin, L. M., Rhoads, G. G., Rich, D. Q., Zhang, J., Bai, Z., Adgate, J. L., Ashley, P.
J., & Lioy, P. J. (2002). "Comparison of techniques to reduce residential lead dust
on carpet and upholstery: the New Jersey assessment of cleaning techniques trial."
*Environmental Health Perspectives*, *110*(12), 1233–1237. https://doi.org/10.1289
/ehp.021101233.

16 "History and Use of Per- and Polyfluoroalkyl Substances (PFAS)," Interstate
Technology and Regulatory Council (ITRC). https://pfas-1.itrcweb.org/fact_sheets_
page/PFAS_Fact_Sheet_History_and_Use_April2020.pdf.

17 Fitten Glenn, A. "Edgy Mama: Toxic toys … research before you buy," Mountainx,
December 6, 2010. https://mountainx.com/arts/art-news/edgy_mama_toxic_toys
_-_research_before_you_buy/.

18 Kuang, J., Abdallah, M. A., & Harrad, S. (2018). "Brominated flame retardants in
black plastic kitchen utensils: Concentrations and human exposure implications."
*The Science of the Total Environment*, *610-611*, 1138–1146. https://doi.org/10.1016/j
.scitotenv.2017.08.173.

19 Samsonek, J., & Puype, F. (2013). "Occurrence of brominated flame retardants in
black thermo cups and selected kitchen utensils purchased on the European market."
*Food Additives & Contaminants. Part A, Chemistry, Analysis, Control, Exposure & Risk
Assessment*, *30*(11), 1976–1986. https://doi.org/10.1080/19440049.2013.829246.

20 Meng T. T. (2014). "Volatile organic compounds of polyethylene vinyl acetate plastic
are toxic to living organisms." *The Journal of Toxicological Sciences*, *39*(5), 795–802.
https://doi.org/10.2131/jts.39.795.

### Chapter 13

1 McMenemy, J. "Water contamination shuts down well at Pease. State raises health
concerns," *Portsmouth Herald*, June 20, 2014. https://www.seacoastonline.com/story
/news/local/portsmouth-herald/2014/06/23/water-contamination-shuts-down
-well/36470148007/.

2 McMenemy, J. "They need to be held accountable," *The Portsmouth Herald*
January 15, 2015. https://www.seacoastonline.com/story/news/local/portsmouth-herald
/2015/01/15/they-need-to-be/33656743007/.

3 McMenemy, J. "Pease water contaminants rattle Seacoast," *Portsmouth Herald*,
Seacoastonline.com, December 30, 2015. https://www.seacoastonline.com/story/news
/local/portsmouth-herald/2015/12/30/pease-water-contaminants-rattle
-seacoast/32810119007/.

4 McMenemy, J. "'My world was crashing down' Amico led fight on Pease water
contamination," *Portsmouth Herald*, December 27, 2015. https://www.seacoastonline
.com/story/news/local/portsmouth-herald/2015/12/27/my-world-was-crashing
/32826186007/.

5   "Average number of hours in the school day and average number of days in the school year for public schools, by state: 2007–08," National Center for Education Statistics. https://nces.ed.gov/surveys/sass/tables/sass0708_035_s1s.asp.

6   Gaffron, P., & Niemeier, D. (2015). "School locations and traffic emissions—environmental (in)justice findings using a new screening method." *International Journal of Environmental Research and Public Health*, *12*(2), 2009–2025. https://doi .org/10.3390/ijerph120202009.

7   Pulimeno, M., Piscitelli, P., Colazzo, S., Colao, A., & Miani, A. (2020). "Indoor air quality at school and students' performance: Recommendations of the UNESCO Chair on Health Education and Sustainable Development & the Italian Society of Environmental Medicine (SIMA)." *Health Promotion Perspectives*, *10*(3), 169–174. https://doi.org/10.34172/hpp.2020.29.

8   Freire, C., Ramos, R., Puertas, R., Lopez-Espinosa, M. J., Julvez, J., Aguilera, I., Cruz, F., Fernandez, M. F., Sunyer, J., & Olea, N. (2010). "Association of traffic-related air pollution with cognitive development in children." *Journal of Epidemiology and Community Health*, *64*(3), 223–228.

9   US EPA O. 2013. *TRI-Listed Chemicals. US EPA.* Available: https://www.epa.gov /toxics-release-inventory-tri-program/tri-listed-chemicals

10  Pianin, E. and Fletcher, M. A. "Many Schools Built Near Toxic Sites, Study Finds," *The Washington Post*, January 21, 2002. https://www.washingtonpost.com/archive /politics/2002/01/21/many-schools-built-near-toxic-sites-study-finds/5c76f67d -bf5f-4fa9-b0a4-39406f477abb/.

11  Gaffron, P., & Niemeier, D. (2015). "School locations and traffic emissions—environmental (in)justice findings using a new screening method." *International Journal of Environmental Research and Public Health*, *12*(2), 2009–2025. https://doi .org/10.3390/ijerph120202009.

12  Heissel, J., Persic, C., Simon, D. "Does Pollution Drive Achievement? The Effect of Traffic Pollution on Academic Performance," National Bureau of Economic Research, January 2019. https://www.nber.org/papers/w25489 WORKING PAPER 25489 DOI 10.3386/w25489.

13  Persico, C., Venator, J. "The Effects of Local Industrial Pollution on Students and Schools," American University School of Public Affairs Research Paper, posted August 7, 2018. https://papers.ssrn.com/sol3/papers.cfm?abstract_id=3218789.

14  Persico, C. & Venator, J., "The Effects of Local Industrial Pollution on Students and Schools," (May 24, 2018). American University School of Public Affairs Research Paper, Available at SSRN: https://ssrn.com/abstract=3218789 or http://dx.doi .org/10.2139/ssrn.3218789.

15  Liu, J., & Schelar, E. (2012). "Pesticide exposure and child neurodevelopment: summary and implications." *Workplace Health & Safety*, *60*(5), 235–243. https://doi .org/10.1177/216507991206000507.

16  Crystal, S. "New Report Shows That More Colleges Have Every Reason to Ditch

Toxic Pesticides," Foodtank.com. https://foodtank.com/news/2022/04/new-report-shows-that-more-colleges-have-every-reason-to-ditch-toxic-pesticides/.

17 Emanuel, G. "Does Your Kid's Classroom Need An Air Purifier? Here's How You Can Make One Yourself," *NPR,* August 26, 2021. https://www.npr.org/sections/back-to-school-live-updates/2021/08/26/1031018250/does-your-kids-classroom-need-an-air-purifier-heres-how-you-can-make-one-yoursel.

18 Lieberman, M. "Air Purifiers, Fans, and Filters: A COVID-19 Explainer for Schools," *Education Week,* October 27, 2020. https://www.edweek.org/leadership/air-purifiers-fans-and-filters-a-covid-19-explainer-for-schools/2020/10.

19 Rubin, T. "A Tale of Two Hydro Flasks: Leaded & Not!" Lead Safe Mama, November 22, 2017. https://tamararubin.com/2017/11/hydro2/.

20 "What Parents Need to Know About Diesel School Buses. If your kids are riding a diesel bus to school, chances are they're being exposed to unacceptable cancer risk." https://www.hpcdfuel.com/wp-content/uploads/2020/01/NRDC_School_Bus_Air_Quality_Report.pdf.

21 Stubbings, W. A., Schreder, E. D., Thomas, M. B., Romanak, K., Venier, M., & Salamova, A. (2018). "Exposure to brominated and organophosphate ester flame retardants in U.S. childcare environments: Effect of removal of flame-retarded nap mats on indoor levels." *Environmental Pollution (Barking, Essex : 1987),* *238,* 1056–1068. https://doi.org/10.1016/j.envpol.2018.03.083.

22 Allayaud, B. "California Makes it Law: Label Toxic Flame Retardants in Furniture," Environmental Working Group, September 30, 2014. https://www.ewg.org/news-insights/news/2014/09/california-makes-it-law-label-toxic-flame-retardants-furniture.

23 Ramadan, L. "Toxic PCBs Festered at This Public School for Eight Years as Students and Teachers Grew Sicker," *ProPublica* and *The Seattle Times,* January 23, 2022. https://www.propublica.org/article/toxic-pcbs-festered-at-this-public-school-for-eight-years-as-students-and-teachers-grew-sicker.

24 Ramadan, L. "Juries award students, parents, teachers $247 million for toxic exposure at Sky Valley Education Center in Monroe," *The Seattle Times,* Nov. 12, 2021. https://www.seattletimes.com/seattle-news/times-watchdog/2nd-multi-million-dollar-verdict-against-monroe-school-for-toxic-exposures/.

25 "How old are America's schools?" National Center for Education Statistics, January 1999. https://nces.ed.gov/pubs99/1999048.pdf.

26 National School Choice Week Team. "The Ultimate Guide to a Public School Transfer (Open Enrollment)," School Choice Week, September 21, 2022. https://schoolchoiceweek.com/public-school-transfer/*

27 Xia, C., Diamond, M. L., Peaslee, G. F., Peng, H., Blum, A., Wang, Z., Shalin, A., Whitehead, H. D., Green, M., Schwartz-Narbonne, H., Yang, D., & Venier, M. (2022). "Per- and Polyfluoroalkyl Substances in North American School Uniforms."

*Environmental Science & Technology*, *56*(19), 13845–13857. https://doi.org/10.1021/acs.est.2c02111.

28  Howard, J. "Soccer players' cancers ignite debate over turf safety," CNN.com, January 27, 2017. https://www.cnn.com/2017/01/27/health/artificial-turf-cancer-study-profile.

29  Jack Bryant. "Happy 19th Birthday!!!" June 10, 2020. https://posthope.org/jack-bryant.

30  International Agency for Research on Cancer (IARC) - Summaries & Evaluations CREOSOTES-(Group 2A) Supplement 7: (1987) (p. 177) https://inchem.org/documents/iarc/suppl7/creosotes.html.

31  Griggs J. L., Rogers K. R., Nelson C., Luxton T., Platten W. E., 3rd, Bradham K. D. "In vitro bioaccessibility of copper azole following simulated dermal transfer from pressure-treated wood." *Sci Total Environ.* 2017 Nov 15;598:413-420. doi: 10.1016/j.scitotenv.2017.03.227. Epub 2017 Apr 25. PMID: 28448933; PMCID: PMC6145065.

32  Reynolds, P., Hurley, S. E., Gunier, R. B., Yerabati, S., Quach, T., & Hertz, A. (2005). "Residential proximity to agricultural pesticide use and incidence of breast cancer in California, 1988-1997." *Environmental Health Perspectives*, *113*(8), 993–1000. https://doi.org/10.1289/ehp.7765.

33  Reynolds, P., Hurley, S. E., Gunier, R. B., Yerabati, S., Quach, T., & Hertz, A. (2005). "Residential proximity to agricultural pesticide use and incidence of breast cancer in California, 1988-1997." *Environmental Health Perspectives*, *113*(8), 993–1000. https://doi.org/10.1289/ehp.7765.

34  Gorpinchenko, I., Nikitin, O., Banyra, O., & Shulyak, A. (2014). "The influence of direct mobile phone radiation on sperm quality." *Central European Journal of Urology*, *67*(1), 65–71. https://doi.org/10.5173/ceju.2014.01.art14.

35  Tsarna, E., Reedijk, M., Birks, L. E., Guxens, M., Ballester, F., Ha, M., Jiménez-Zabala, A., Kheifets, L., Lertxundi, A., Lim, H. R., Olsen, J., González Safont, L., Sudan, M., Cardis, E., Vrijheid, M., Vrijkotte, T., Huss, A., & Vermeulen, R. (2019). "Associations of Maternal Cell-Phone Use During Pregnancy With Pregnancy Duration and Fetal Growth in 4 Birth Cohorts." *American Journal of Epidemiology*, *188*(7), 1270–1280. https://doi.org/10.1093/aje/kwz092.

36  Karuserci Ö.K., Çöl N., Demirel C. "May electromagnetic field exposure during pregnancy have a negative effect on anthropometric measurements of the newborn?" *Cukurova Med. J.* 2019;44(1):290–295.

37  Takei R., Nagaoka T., Nishino K., Saito K., Watanabe S., Takahashi M. "Specific absorption rate and temperature increase in pregnant women at 13, 18, and 26 weeks of gestation due to electromagnetic wave radiation from a smartphone." *IEICE Commun. Express.* 2018;7(6):212–217.

38  Saadia Z. (2018). "Impact of Maternal Obesity and Mobile Phone Use on Fetal Cardiotocography Pattern." *Open Access Macedonian Journal of Medical Sciences*, *6*(10), 1813–1817. https://doi.org/10.3889/oamjms.2018.405.

39 Li, D. K., Chen, H., Ferber, J. R., Odouli, R., & Quesenberry, C. (2017). "Exposure to Magnetic Field Non-Ionizing Radiation and the Risk of Miscarriage: A Prospective Cohort Study." *Scientific Reports*, *7*(1), 17541. https://doi.org/10.1038/s41598-017-16623-8.

40 "FACT SHEET: Inflation Reduction Act Advances Environmental Justice," The White House, August 17, 2022. https://www.whitehouse.gov/briefing-room/statements releases/2022/08/17/fact-sheet-inflation-reduction-act-advances-environmental -justice/.

41 Kamenetz, A. "There's a lot of new federal money for greening K-12 education. This is how schools could use it: Here are seven steps schools can take to claim their piece of the clean, green pie," *The Hechinger Report,* December 20, 2022. https://hechinger report.org/column-theres-a-lot-of-new-federal-money-for-greening-k-12-education -this-is-how-schools-could-use-it/.

42 Lieberman, M. "What Does the Inflation Reduction Act Mean for K-12 Schools?" *Government Tech*, August 3, 2022. https://www.govtech.com/education/k-12/what -does-the-inflation-reduction-act-mean-for-k-12-schools.

### Chapter 14

1 Darom, N. "What It's Like to Discover You're Non-binary," *Haaretz*, April 18, 2017. https://www.haaretz.com/us-news/2017-08-18/ty-article-magazine/.premium /what-its-like-to-discover-youre-non-binary/0000017f-e307-d9aa-afff-fb5ff42a0000.

2 Ndebele, K., Graham, B., & Tchounwou, P. B. (2010). "Estrogenic activity of coume-strol, DDT, and TCDD in human cervical cancer cells." *International Journal of Environmental Research and Public Health*, *7*(5), 2045–2056. https://doi.org/10.3390 /ijerph7052045.

3 Zhong, L., Xiang, X., Lu, W., Zhou, P., & Wang, L. (2013). "Interference of xen-oestrogen o,p'-DDT on the action of endogenous estrogens at environmentally real-istic concentrations." *Bulletin of Environmental Contamination and Toxicology*, *90*(5), 591–595. https://doi.org/10.1007/s00128-013-0976-9.

4 Swaab, D. F., & Garcia-Falgueras, A. (2009). "Sexual differentiation of the human brain in relation to gender identity and sexual orientation." *Functional Neurology*, *24*(1), 17–28.

5 Dixon, S. "Number of monthly active Facebook users worldwide as of 4th quarter 2022 (in millions)," *Statista*, Feb 13, 2023. https://www.statista.com/statistics/264810 /number-of-monthly-active-facebook-users-worldwide/.

6 Griggs,B. "Facebook goes beyond 'male' and 'female' with new gender options," CNN.com, February 13, 2014. https://www.cnn.com/2014/02/13/tech/social-media /facebook-gender-custom/index.html.

7 Ball, A. L. "In All-Gender Restrooms, the Signs Reflect the Times," *The New York Times*, Nov. 5, 2015. https://www.nytimes.com/2015/11/08/style/transgender-restroom -all-gender.html.

8  Rider, G. N., McMorris, B. J., Gower, A. L., Coleman, E., & Eisenberg, M. E. (2018). "Health and Care Utilization of Transgender and Gender Nonconforming Youth: A Population-Based Study." *Pediatrics*, *141*(3), e20171683. https://doi.org/10.1542/peds.2017-1683.

9  Tanner, Lindsey. "Not just boy and girl; more teens identify as transgender," Associated Press, February 4, 2018. https://apnews.com/article/health-north-america-lifestyle-il-state-wire-us-news-02e14dcaba1f44af8202d390794f8717.

10 Kaltiala-Heino, R., Bergman, H., Työläjärvi, M., & Frisén, L. (2018). "Gender dysphoria in adolescence: current perspectives." *Adolescent Health, Medicine and Therapeutics*, *9*, 31–41. https://doi.org/10.2147/AHMT.S135432.

11 Kinsey, A. C., Pomeroy, W. R., & Martin, C. E. (2003). "Sexual behavior in the human male. 1948." *American Journal of Public Health*, *93*(6), 894–898. https://doi.org/10.2105/ajph.93.6.894.

12 Meanley, S., Haberlen, S. A., Okafor, C. N., Brown, A., Brennan-Ing, M., Ware, D., Egan, J. E., Teplin, L. A., Bolan, R. K., Friedman, M. R., & Plankey, M. W. (2020). "Lifetime Exposure to Conversion Therapy and Psychosocial Health Among Midlife and Older Adult Men Who Have Sex With Men." *The Gerontologist*, *60*(7), 1291–1302. https://doi.org/10.1093/geront/gnaa069.

13 "Gender Dysphoria Diagnosis History," American Psychiatric Association. https://www.psychiatry.org/psychiatrists/diversity/education/transgender-and-gender-nonconforming-patients/gender-dysphoria-diagnosis.

14 "LGBTQ definitions," University of Colorado Center for Inclusion and Social Change. https://www.colorado.edu/cisc/resources/trans-queer/lgbtq-definitions.

15 2023 legislative session The ACLU is tracking 452 anti-LGBTQ bills in the U.S., American Civil Liberties Union. https://www.aclu.org/legislative-attacks-on-lgbtq-rights.

16 Lavietes, M. & Ramos, E. "Nearly 240 anti-LGBTQ bills filed in 2022 so far, most of them targeting trans people. The annual number of anti-LGBTQ bills to have been filed has skyrocketed over the past several years, from 41 in 2018 to 238 in less than three months of this year," *NBC News,* March 20, 2022. https://www.nbcnews.com/nbc-out/out-politics-and-policy/nearly-240-anti-lgbtq-bills-filed-2022-far-targeting-trans-people-rcna20418.

## Chapter 15

1  Schlanger, Z. "KILLER SMOG: The story of 26 sudden deaths in 1948 is a bleak reminder of why America needs clean air laws," *Quartz*, November 1, 2017. https://qz.com/1117029/the-sudden-death-of-26-people-in-a-tiny-american-town-on-halloween-weekend-shows-the-bleak-reality-of-life-before-clean-air-laws.

2  This event led to the first large-scale epidemiological investigation of an environmental health disaster in the United States.

3  Frazier, R. "Rachel Carson Trail Near Pittsburgh Has a New Feature: A Fracking

Well," *The Allegheny Front*, June 22, 2018. https://www.alleghenyfront.org/rachel -carson-trail-near-pittsburgh-has-a-new-feature-a-fracking-well/.

4   Sisk, A. "Young Activists Want to Make Climate Change a Political Priority. Here's Their Plan," *The Allegheny Front*, July 20, 2018. https://www.alleghenyfront.org /young-activists-want-to-make-climate-change-a-political-priority-and-they-have-a -plan-to-do-just-that/.

5   Lindwall, C. "The Student Activist Fighting Pittsburgh's Dirty Industry," NRDC.org, May 23, 2019. https://www.nrdc.org/stories/student-activist-fighting-pittsburghs-dirty -industry.

6   Ibid.

7   Davidson, J. "How to Raise an Environmentalist," Natural Resources Defense Council, April 19, 2018. https://www.nrdc.org/stories/how-raise-environmentalist.

8   USDA Agricultural Marketing Service. "Local Food Directories: Community Supported Agriculture (CSA) Directory," US Department of Agriculture. https: //www.ams.usda.gov/local-food-directories/csas.

9   Frack, K. "10 Cities Pushing the Bounds of Community Gardening," *Seedstock,* April 18, 2016. https://seedstock.com/2016/04/18/10-cites-pushing-the-bounds-of-community -gardening/.

10   "Southeast Conservation Corps Women's Crew," YouTube.com https://www.youtube .com/watch?v=XkFHOMDbRGc.

11   Kuo, F. E., & Taylor, A. F. (2004). "A potential natural treatment for attention-deficit /hyperactivity disorder: evidence from a national study." *American Journal of Public Health*, *94*(9), 1580–1586. https://doi.org/10.2105/ajph.94.9.1580.

# Author's Note

There will always be honest differences of opinion when it comes to science and product ratings—especially in the evaluation and interpretation of information about short-and long-term health and environmental effects arising from chemical exposures and pollution. This book represents my views on product safety based on facts obtained from a variety of sources.

In evaluating foods and consumer products, I have endeavored to be thorough and conscientious in the review of the information provided by local, state, federal, and international agencies, industry, published, peer-reviewed studies in the scientific literature, news reports, and independent analytical laboratory results the Healthy Living Foundation (HLF) has acquired in its advocacy of the consumer's right to know about hidden chemical toxins.

Anyone who knows of data that may alter the evaluation of the foods and products reviewed in this book is encouraged to make this information available to the author by writing in care of Skyhorse Publishing, 307 West 36th Street, 11th Floor, New York, NY 10018 (212) 643-681 or via online at https://www. skyhorsepublishing.com/contact-us/.

Furthermore, I welcome readers' comments about foods, product brands, areas of concern that may have been overlooked, and your own personal stories of hidden toxic exposures. I look forward to hearing from you.

# Acknowledgments

I could never have written *Raising Healthy Kids* without the help of countless persons.

I thank the many activist parents who shared their own personal inspiring narratives. Never before have the stories of so many antitoxic activists been gathered under one cover.

Salinas, California, has a special place in my heart. I want to extend my gratitude to Oscar Ramos, the second-grade teacher and parent, who shared his own experiences with me as a labor-camp child; elementary school math teacher Joshua Ezekiel who guided me from one school to another; CHAMACOS youths Daisy Gallardo, Jessica Cabrera, and Stephanie Mayo-Burgos who offer so much hope for a brighter future; Drs. Brenda Eskenazi, Kim Harley, and their colleagues at UC Berkeley's Center for Environmental Research and Children's Health who worked with the teens of Salinas to put together the many informative studies taking place there, in so doing, helped to elevate a group of kids to extraordinary achievements at such young ages; and the many farmers and farmworkers who bring us our daily bread; for all, I wish a safe and healthy life.

Mel Coleman, Jr., of Saguache Colorado, and Albert Straus, of Marshall, California, shared their stories of regenerative agriculture and thriving during difficult economic times with innovations that nurture the earth and honor our farm animals.

Dr. John Meeker, Senior Associate Dean for Research, University of Michigan School of Public Health, has advised our nonprofit group Healthy Living Foundation on matters of environmental exposures and public health and contributed to a fundamental understanding of the dangers of low-level exposures to the pesticide carbaryl as well as acrylamide, phthalates, and other chemical toxins.

Thank you to Angela Sutherland and Evelyn Rusli for bringing safe, healthy, and fresh organic baby foods to consumers.

Stephanie Mero, of Orlando, Florida, shared her beauty-industry story and offers hope to hundreds of thousands of persons that they can do what they love without toxic chemicals—and have a healthy family, too.

Michael Hickey and Loreen Hackett of Hoosick Falls, New York, Sharon C. Lavigne of St. James Parish, Louisiana, Robert Taylor, of nearby Reserve, Brenda Hampton of Lawrence County, Alabama, Andrea Amico, of Portsmouth, New Hampshire, Stel Bailey from Cocoa, Florida, and Dianne and Anaïs Peterson, of O'Hara Township, Pennsylvania, deserve medals of honor for their activism in protecting their communities. My friend Susan Wind deserves special recognition for protecting the citizens of Mooresville, North Carolina, while simultaneously uniting activists from across the nation when they gathered at the historic September 20, 2020 "We're Here Too" national demonstration in Washington, D.C. calling for an end to the toxic poisoning of communities across the land.

I am grateful for the personal courage, clarity, and shared wisdom of Mere Abrams, L.C.S.W., and Dana Beyer, M.D, who've helped to bring light to gender identity.

Early on, when there was barely a hint of *Raising Healthy Kids*, Joe Perry of Perry Literary Agency believed in my work, and I will always be grateful.

Kevin Wood, senior editor at *Good Men Project*, championed publishing my investigative reports that are the basis for *Raising Healthy Kids*.

I am thankful to Michael Pietsch, Natalie Chapman, and John Oakes whose passion for my work led to *Diet for a Poisoned Planet, Safe Shopper's Bible*, and *Safe Trip to Eden*, respectively. Thank you to Madeleine Morel and William Clark for representing these works.

I would disappoint my kids if I didn't offer homage to Rufi and Flynn, our black-and-white border collies, and our twenty-year-old leopard gecko who have been our family therapy and taught us to be kind and gentle.

Nicole Frail, my editor, and Tony Lyons, the president of Skyhorse Publishing, championed *Raising Healthy Kids* and provided me the time and space to turn in and produce a quality work.

Mark Chimsky is my longtime editorial consultant. I couldn't have written this story without him.

Daniella Bordeaux's interest in the development of this book and consistent encouragement helped to develop these words into this song.

# Index